treating
the school age
stutterer
a guide for clinicians

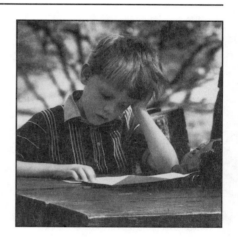

by CARL W. DELL, JR.

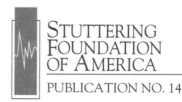

STUTTERING
FOUNDATION
OF AMERICA

PUBLICATION NO. 14

Published by

Stuttering Foundation of America
Formerly Speech Foundation of America
P. O. Box 11749
Memphis, Tennessee 38111

Library of Congress Catalog No. 79-67284
ISBN-0-933388-11-X

FIRST PRINTING–1979
SECOND PRINTING–1983
THIRD PRINTING–1986
FOURTH PRINTING–1989
FIFTH PRINTING–1991
SIXTH PRINTING–1994

The Stuttering Foundation of America is a non-profit charitable organization dedicated to the prevention and treatment of stuttering. Contributions are tax-deductible and help us continue our work.

To the Public School Clinician

This book describes how you can work effectively with young stutterers. This information was obtained through an extensive program of study, testing and research carried on for several years. The author, a public school clinician, participated in this program after special training with Dr. Charles Van Riper, considered one of the world's foremost authorities on the therapy of stuttering.

Originally funded by the Stuttering Foundation of America, the author worked as a stuttering specialist cooperating with the school clinicians in the Grand Rapids, Michigan, metropolitan area with a school population of around 120,000. Special thanks for the results still being achieved in this program are due the clinicians in Kent County with whom he works and for the cooperation of Joe Noorthoek, the assistant superintendent for special education in that district.

These suggestions and recommendations make quite interesting reading. And we believe that the utilization of this information cannot help but make your efforts on behalf of the young stutterer more effective and rewarding.

Malcolm Fraser

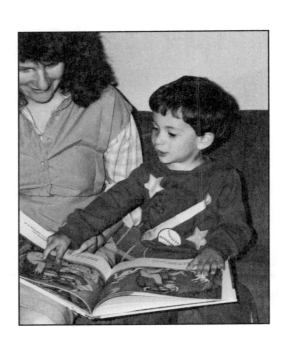

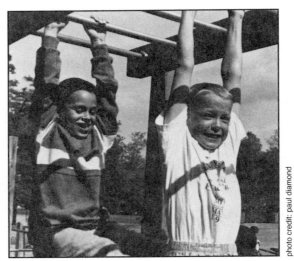

photo credit: paul diamond

Introduction

Several attempts have been made to make stuttering therapy easier for the school clinician and some of us have found success using these easier methods. If you are one of the latter you are truly blessed because many others have found only failure and frustration. Some of us have used a new method successfully on one stuttering child only to find that when we try it on another we fail miserably. And there are those of us who have come to mistrust anything that tries to simplify the problem of treating the young stutterer. Stuttering seems so complex that easy ways somehow seem fraudulent and sometimes they are.

Solving complex problems with simple solutions has rarely been effective. Take the subject of weight loss for example. How many books have claimed to provide a quick and easy way to lose weight! While there always are a few ardent followers who have had success by using the new, easy diets or methods, most who try them end in failure. Then they reach out to grab another fad diet and the cycle begins again. Only consistent work and great determination seems to create any real success. So too with stuttering. Most children who stutter will have to endure some frustration and effort to overcome their stuttering. Perhaps this is not as bad as it sounds. All of us grow through adversity and we usually discover that the hard fought battles are those which bring the greatest reward. No, the treatment of stuttering is rarely easy so it is understandable that many public school clinicians dread working with children who possess the problem.

Some are reluctant to work with stutterers because they feel they cannot really understand the disorder. School clinicians often ask if any normal speaking clinician can ever truly identify with a stuttering child? We would reply that all of us have known frustration, anxiety and embarrassment, and since all of us share some measure of human frailty we can empathize with the stutterer's feelings well enough to establish the necessary working relationship.

Another way to get better understanding is to learn how the young client stutters. By using a tape recorder you can get some recorded samples of his abnormal speech and then, after the child leaves, you can try to imitate the stuttering, using a large mirror to mimic the facial and body gestures he has shown. This along with

7

your clinical training and academic knowledge about the nature of stuttering should enable you to identify enough with the young stutterer to help him.

But it is often difficult to work with a stuttering child in the schools. The author knows personally the kind of conditions in which most of you must work. We public school clinicians live different professional lives than the rest of our colleagues. We may not find a room available and must use a storage room or the hallway. Or we may have trouble even getting the child out of his classroom for often it seems that teachers are always doing special projects when we need to see him.* But the major difficulty we have in working with stutterers is our lack of time, experience and faith. This is what one school clinician told us: "When there are 75 other children to see twice a week, plus the increasing amount of paper work that I am now being forced to handle, it is difficult to give any one child enough of my time. And the stutterer takes a lot of time and work. Also I don't see many stutterers in any one year since articulation and language problems are my major concern."

During a recent state convention a group of school clinicians were pouring out their frustrations nearly as fast as they were pouring down an assorted array of beverages at a nearby watering hole. The subject turned to stuttering: "You know," said one young clinician, "They make it sound so easy but I really dread having a stutterer. I feel so fraudulent. The parents, teacher and the child himself are always coming to me for help thinking I have all the answers to the stuttering problem. It's hard to pretend I'm confident when I'm really not."

"Yes, I know the feeling," said an older clinician, "I have seen quite a few stutterers over the years but still I don't feel very competent. I have had several dramatically unsuccessful cases. Sometimes I dread getting another one."

Certainly these clinicians are not alone. Most of our public school colleagues could make similar confessions and so could our fellow workers in clinical settings.

It is natural for clinicians to have these fears about their stuttering clients. Stuttering is a complicated and perplexing disorder. Our speech libraries are full of books about it but still we know so little. Although the clinician may have been trained in one of our best

---

*During the course of this book we will use the masculine pronouns when referring to stuttering clients and female pronouns for speech clinicians.

institutions she still feels inadequate in trying to help a young stutterer. A colleague summed it up this way: "I know quite a lot about stuttering but little about working with a stuttering client."

We could list other reasons why working with a stutterer is difficult but we must remember that we know more about stuttering than anyone else associated with the child. Who else can help him? Who else has the background we have — even if it isn't enough? In trying to be honest and truthful we are quick to point out our inadequacies and feelings of failure but seldom do we mention or are we praised for the skillful way we interact with troubled children. We know how to give these children a feeling of worth, and dignity. They can find acceptance, warmth and understanding in our room. In us they will find someone who listens even if they stutter, someone who won't wince or reject, someone who wants to help.

So let us take pride in our professional abilities for we have much to offer a child that he cannot get elsewhere. These children need all the help we can provide and we may give them more than we think. Certainly the only way we can gain experience and improve our skills is by working with stutterers, not by avoiding them.

Let me tell you about some of my own personal feelings as a young stutterer going to speech class, for I have been on both sides of the therapy room table. Although my stuttering was not cured during my school years, the school clinicians did accomplish several very important things. They provided a place where I could come and talk, where no one would laugh at me or scorn me, where I felt free to communicate even if I did stutter. What a great feeling that was! My dog was the only other living creature with whom I felt that way. Here was a place where I could learn something about my stuttering, that mysterious thing that no one else ever mentioned. I needed a safe place where I could touch it and confront it. All of these benefited me a great deal as a young boy. My public school clinicians didn't cure me but they were sorely needed and I believe these experiences laid the foundation for my eventual success. Indeed, I'm certain that, without this early therapy background, my therapy as an adult would have been much more difficult. But most valuable of all was the gift of caring. They cared! I was made to feel some worth as a human being despite my stuttering. Because of this experience, stuttering did not destroy my self-concept the way it does in many young stutterers. The caring and warmth I received from my school clinicians helped me stay together as a person.

Although I remain grateful to all the public school clinicians who helped me, I believe that much more can be done than they were able to do. Most importantly, they should have tried to reverse the progressive course of stuttering. Unfortunately too many borderline and mild stutterers become severe, confirmed stutterers and we feel that the public school clinician can prevent this. There seems to be at least two reasons why so many stutterers get worse during their school years. The first is that they get no professional help in the early stages of their stuttering, and the second is that the clinician hasn't been trained to provide the necessary methods for preventing its abnormal growth. It is our belief that the key to the problem of stuttering is early intervention so that the progressive growth of the disorder can be reversed. It is our experience that if this can be done early enough, stuttering can be cured.

The major purpose of this book will be to present some practical ways in which the public school clinician might intervene with young stutterers to accomplish this goal. Although we have successfully been able to achieve it we are sure that others have found some success using other approaches. It is not our purpose to debate the effectiveness of different methods. Our present goal is simply to convince clinicians of the importance of scheduling these young stutterers rather than putting them on hold. The treatment of any human ailment is easier and more effective when it is begun during the onset of the disorder. We are convinced that this is true of stuttering.

For organizational purposes the author has reluctantly divided young stutterers into three groups: Borderline, Mild and Confirmed. Although this has helped to organize the material it may give the impression that we group stutterers. We do not! All young stutterers fall somewhere along a severity scale and fluctuate within it and in practice we make no attempt to categorize them. A child's severity is simply one of several dimensions we use in designing his individual therapy. It, along with the child's basic intelligence, his social maturity and age, will tell us how direct we will attack his stuttering.

The author also feels a need to explain our use of the term "clinician". Those of us in the public schools have labored under a variety of titles. We have been called "speech teacher", "speech therapist", "speech pathologist", and now "speech and language pathologists". However we will use the term "clinician" hereafter because of its general acceptance in our field. This is done merely to provide uniformity in our presentation and not to take a stand on the issue of professional titles.

The Borderline Stutterer

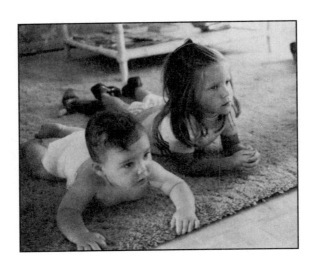

The Borderline Stutterer

One of the questions school clinicians often ask is when they should start working with a young stutterer? They don't want to begin too soon because they think the child might outgrow it in a year or two. Some of this reluctance comes from feeling professionally inadequate but some clinicians are truly afraid of making the child worse. As one put it: "If I draw attention to the problem isn't it possible the child might become morbid and develop more advanced forms of stuttering?

Theoretically it seems possible that a child might get worse because he has been taken out of his room for speech. He may consider this as being an indication that he is inferior or abnormal. If then he tries harder to speak perfectly his disfluencies may increase and he may become frustrated and fearful. Although this seems logical we have never seen it happen in reality, never once! Perhaps if the clinician's attitude toward the child were negative or if she shows an aversion to stuttering when it occurs then the stuttering might get worse, but our experience has been that most clinicians are loving, gentle people who accept and understand the child's stuttering. Such attitudes will not make the stuttering worse. Also, we must remember that many people have already been critical of the child's stuttering. People often claim that the child is completely unaware of his stuttering, but they are usually wrong. In our first meeting he usually tells us he stutters. It may be something as innocent as this: "I know my Mom doesn't like it because she often looks down when I do it." Usually, when the child is taken out of class it isn't the first time that attention has been drawn to his stuttering.

Another thing that school clinicians worry about is doing something wrong during therapy that will cause the child to get worse. Certainly we all make mistakes, but this is no reason to avoid seeing the child. Because of their resiliency, children are rarely affected for very long. If the clinician is alert to changes in the client's behavior she can always adjust her therapy accordingly. With each client our goals can be reached not only by following different routes but also by moving at different speeds. So let us have confidence in our abilities. Any good clinician will make a mistake occasionally but she is quick to recognize it and make appropriate adjustments.

It is also true a child in therapy may get worse for reasons that have nothing to do with you. He may be having difficulties at home, e.g., his parents may be having trouble getting along, or they may have made some decisions that the child resents, or he may be having trouble with his siblings. A colleague told of calling the home of a young beginning stutterer after she noticed a drastic increase in his stuttering. "Yesterday," the mother told her, "Billy got terribly excited when I bought him that Spiderman costume for Halloween and he stuttered a lot. Then his dad wouldn't allow him to go out Halloween night because he had left his bike out the night before. And he had a fight with his brother that he lost. All in all he had a tough day."

All sorts of experiences can provoke an increase in stuttering. The child may be having trouble with his peers. The children in school or in the neighborhood may be giving him a hard time. Children often live in one crisis after another but fortunately they rebound quickly. So there's no need for the clinician to blame herself for any temporary increase in disfluency. Any particular stuttering child may be affected enough by any of these outside conflicts to cause his speech to get worse.

Another question clinicians ask is how to decide when a child is merely normally disfluent and when he is stuttering badly enough to require our services. Clinicians who take only the severe stutterers may never need to make this distinction but if we are to prevent stuttering we must serve the borderline stutterers too. We do not believe that any danger exists of turning a normally disfluent child into a stutterer if the clinician works with him appropriately. The indirect form of therapy that we advocate can be beneficial for both the stutterer or the normally disfluent child. If your therapy sessions are relaxed and nonthreatening you should have little fear of any unfortunate consequences. Indeed, we have often had a teacher ask us to take other students for therapy after we were fortunate enough to have some success with one of their stuttering pupils. When we asked if the child stuttered the teacher said, "No, but you helped little Johnny so much, in more ways than just his stuttering, that I'm sure that this troubled child would profit too." Any child will benefit from your warm attention and understanding. Few children get enough friendly attention in their lives and certainly some of them need more of it.

So we need have no fears about enrolling a child in therapy who might or might not be a real stutterer. Instead of ignoring these disfluent children or putting them on hold, it is often wise to enroll them if only to provide time for further evaluation. We need this time and contact. All of us have been fooled by children whom we thought were normally disfluent only to find, after a few sessions of some indirect therapy, that they were genuine stutterers. Some stutterers have the ability to hide their problem with great skill. They have practiced hiding the stuttering from their parents and classmates and know therefore that the speech teacher is an exposure threat to them. Moreover, some don't want to admit even to themselves that they are stutterers. They reason that if the speech teacher finds out they stutter then all the other kids will know about it too and then they will be teased unmercifully. These and other fears will often make the young stutterer generate that extra bit of adrenalin to enable him for the moment to speak very well. Even severe adult stutterers can occasionally be fluent at times of great stress. We have found some young stutterers who have learned how to avoid and substitute with such skill that they are able to fool even an experienced clinician. But if we see a child for two to four sessions the child's defenses will usually break down and he simply cannot keep up the pretense of being fluent for that long. One of our colleagues related this story:

> She had recently been assigned to a new school district which had had a high turnover of speech clinicians in recent years. Late in the fall she received a call from a mother who insisted that her seventh grade boy was stuttering worse than ever and would she do something about it. The mother told of her frustrations with other clinicians in the past. "They always refused to help Mike because they said he didn't stutter. I just wish they could hear him at home sometime."
>
> The clinician saw the boy and although he seemed somewhat shy and nervous he talked without any stuttering at all. She asked Mike's teachers and they said they hadn't noticed any stuttering. Reluctantly she called the home and told the mother that the boy seemed to be doing fine at school. The mother was angry and seemed desperate. The clinician was curious. Perhaps a parent conference would yield some answers. Perhaps the parents were being unduly perfectionistic.
>
> When the parents came the clinician was again impressed by their earnestness and concern. Their descriptions of Mike's stuttering gave a picture of a severe, confirmed stutterer so she agreed to see Mike once a week.

During the first two sessions Mike was as fluent as ever and, as he came to like his clinician, he began talking more. It was during the next session that Mike's protective wall began to crumble. The clinician noticed some mild stuttering although of course she didn't react to it. Soon Mike began stuttering enough so that the clinician brought it to his attention. They began to discuss his speech. When Mike saw that she was interested rather than corrective he seemed to breathe a sigh of relief. What followed was more stuttering than the clinician had ever heard.

Mike had spent a lifetime in fear and hiding, always trying to protect his stuttering from the world. Trying to hide it from his parents was just too much work but he could hide it from others although not without a great expense of effort and strain. He truly needed help.

It is wise also to spread your diagnostic sessions with a disfluent child over a period of time such as once a week for several weeks because many young stutterers have cycles in which they alternate between fluency and stuttering. Perhaps your one session with him occurred during his fluent cycle. If so, once again, you may have seen a false picture. Missing a real stutterer can be professionally more embarrassing than working with a normally disfluent child will ever be. Generally if you see a child for three or four sessions and no real stuttering occurs it is wise to tell the teacher that the child does seem to be slow in developing normal fluency but that in your opinion there is no real reason for concern. But you should also tell her that you are therefore not going to continue working with him but that if she, the teacher, notices any change for the worse in his speech she should let you know and you will be glad to see him immediately. By following this policy the teacher will feel that you have shown an interest in her problems. You have taken the time to see one of her children and to study him intensively. This can only add to your professional credibility in her eyes and in the opinion of her colleagues. Conversely, if you see a child only once and report that he is just normally disfluent or that you feel he will outgrow any disfluecies and that child continues to stutter in the classroom under stress you will have lost the respect of that teacher. She will feel that you have not taken the necessary time with the child she has referred. So it is wise to conduct a thorough evaluation when these children are placed in your hands.

Group Placement for Further Evaluation

Many clinicians have occasionally put these borderline stutterers in articulation or language groups, using their normal articulation and language as models for the others. This gives the clinician a good chance to observe the child over a period of time and since the sessions are casual and low key, the borderline stutterer is made to feel comfortable and under no threat. Often if he is quite advanced in articulation or language and therefore able to excel in the group, this experience may actually help him be more fluent. Clinicians have found that such a group encounter is an excellent vehicle for determining if the child is really a stutterer and sometimes this group therapy has actually helped him overcome his mild stuttering.

For other children this placement in articulation and language groups may show the clinician that real stuttering is developing. If so, and if you need to take him out of the group for individual sessions the prior placement in the articulation or language group may make the transition easier.

Another problem arises, however, when the disfluent child also has a real articulation problem. Putting too much pressure on his articulation errors may bring on more stuttering by creating fears of certain sounds. While you can still enroll him in the group you should watch him closely so that you can quickly determine whether your work on his articulation is causing him more difficulty. If so, he should be taken out of the group and seen individually unless you can find ways to keep the stuttering from increasing. Sometimes you can do this by reducing your demands or by working on an easier sound.

Another question that some have raised is how one explains to the other children the disfluent child's membership in the articulation or language group. This is another theoretical problem which rarely causes our clinicians much trouble in practice. Children in an articulation or language group just don't seem to notice that our disfluent child is any different. If the clinician makes a simple statement like: "Johnny sometimes has trouble when he says his words. He may get stuck on a word sometimes like this, "I-I-I." We find children to be very accepting. They seem to realize that mastering disfluency errors, like conquering their articulation, is just a part of learning to talk better.

Some clinicians might fear to do this outward imitation of the child's disfluencies. However since clinicians often demonstrate errors in articulation therapy while teaching phonemic discrimination, why avoid the practice with stuttering? Children seem to accept our casual imitation and identification of stuttering behavior without any reaction at all. If occasionally they laugh, it is no different from the laugh that comes when we imitate a defective 's' sound in front of other children. Why can't we do the same with a disfluency? The reason that stuttering has such a stigma attached to it is because many of us are reluctant to confront the child with his stuttering. Most of the adults in the child's life have tried to either correct the child or to ignore the disfluency. The little child often needs straight-forward talk if he is to accept his problem as a problem. The other children tease him about it on the playground but no one has ever explained to him what he is doing. No wonder stuttering is so unpleasant to a child.

There are two important things that we need to remember when talking with the child about his stuttering behaviors or disfluencies. One is to be casual in our approach, to show that we are not shocked by stuttering, and to indicate that we have seen such things before. Talking for some of us is difficult and some of us have a harder time than others in learning how to do it well.

Second, it is important for the clinician to be able occasionally to demonstrate the child's disfluency, to put it into her own mouth without being upset. This does many positive things for the child. It shows him that he is not the only one who can talk like he does. It shows him that others can stutter at will, that it need not be involuntary, that stuttering isn't some kind of curse or disease. In the context of such clinician calmness and honesty he gradually comes to the realization that stuttering need not be feared, that it isn't a shameful thing. Up to this time he has often felt that talking well or poorly is governed purely by luck or chance, that stuttering is mysterious and unacceptable. Moreover the clinician's confrontation and acceptance of the problem through sharing the behaviors often opens the door to feelings that may have been previously repressed. How quickly shame and guilt begin in the young stutterer when stuttering is unmentionable. Like wetting the bed, it is something no one discusses in public. If the child has begun to feel some shame and guilt, occasionally putting his stuttering calmly into your own mouth will surely help to change those dangerous feelings.

Obtaining a Differential Diagnosis

Even after enrolling a student for therapy we always continue to evaluate him for we are still not sure whether he needs our help.

What is it that we are looking for to help us determine whether the child is stuttering or is normally disfluent, or getting better or getting worse? What are some of the cues that should help you decide whether to work with him intensively on a regular schedule? There are many references in the literature that can help you make this decision but each clinician, over a period of time begins to develop her own set of criteria. We have found that the following list has been useful to us:

Guidelines for Differentiating a Stutterer from a Nonfluent Child

Speech Behavior Indicating Risk of Becoming a Stutterer
1. Facial tremors caused by excessive tension.
2. Speaks cautiously.
3. Speaks very rapidly, almost compulsively.
4. Speaks too loudly or softly.
5. Evidences of struggle and tension while speaking.
6. Blocks the airflow.
7. Raises the pitch or volume during disfluencies.
8. Accompanying body movements during disfluencies.
9. Signs of embarrassment while speaking.
10. Uneven repetitions.
11. Use of the schwa vowel on his repetitions.
12. Many repetitions (5 or more) during a word.
13. Stops in the middle of a word, backs up and starts over.
14. Evidence of avoiding certain words.
15. More than one disfluency during a sentence.

Non Speech Behavior Indicating Risk of Becoming a Stutterer
1. Shyness, looks away especially when he is disfluent.
2. Low self concept.
3. Other nervous habits, e.g., nail biting, bed wetting, hyperactivity.
4. Poor socialization skills.
5. Evidences of depression and sadness.
6. Worry.

This of course does not mean that all shy, disfluent children are stutterers but when a child shows a large number of these behaviors we should be concerned. These lists are just one of the tools to help us make our diagnostic judgments. Unlike the adult it is very difficult to categorize any young stutterer because the stuttering is so variable and inconsistent. Criteria are hard to define and most of us have learned to rely on our subjective impressions. The experienced clinician depends on her past experiences in making a differential diagnosis. Let it be said here that we are not against objective facts and close observation, but it is hard at times to make judgments concerning the young stutterer solely on the basis of textbook criteria. A good clinician should trust her feelings as well as her objective observations. Naturally any decision arrived at through subjective means should always be questioned and tested and every decision should be subject to reappraisal and change.

Observe a Variety of Speaking Situations

Before deciding whether a child is showing stuttering behaviors it is also wise to observe the child in as many different speaking situations as possible. We have listened at the door or from a corner of the room while our client has participated in the "show and tell" activities of his classroom and we have learned much while observing him at play during recess. Although it is important to visit with teachers during recess it is also good to spend some time watching our client on the playground. This can even be done at times from the window of the school building as we drink that well earned cup of coffee. Although we can't hear the child we can watch him interacting with the others. Is he a leader or a follower? Is he a real part of a group or does he seem to be hanging around the fringes? Does he stay around the supervising teacher or play with younger children? What are the personalities of his closest playmates? To gather more specific speech information we have ventured directly onto the playground, accompanying the supervising teacher or wandering near enough to our client's classmates to hear them talking. Most of the time the children seem oblivious to our presence. If they should question us about being there we tell them that we wanted to watch them play and needed some fresh air too. They don't question this and quickly return to their play. At times we have felt almost invisible for children play with such intensity and concentration they soon forget we are there. Thus we have often been able to get a good idea of our client's speech while playing with his peers.

Again, it is useful to observe the child when he is talking with his teacher. After sharing our desire with the teacher beforehand we walk around the room talking to the other children, finding out what projects they are working on. Then, when we get close enough to be able to hear our client the teacher goes over and talks with him. She may, for example, question him about a picture he is drawing. Although we may seem to be talking with another youngster we can also be listening with the other ear to our client. At times we have made such arrangements to hear our client talking with the janitor, principal or his parents. These and other observations can be arranged occasionally without much trouble. Too often only the client's speech in the therapy room is considered in evaluating his fluency and this may be quite different from his speech in other situations. The more situations we can observe the better we will be able to understand and help him.

Also, we need to find out his ability to speak while using different types of communication. Too often we tend only to converse with our client. While this occasionally can be adequate it often doesn't give us enough information about the child's speech. He may be fluent in one type of communication but have trouble in others. We may, for instance, have him describe in detail all of the things he sees in our room (description). We can have him explain how his favorite game is played (explanation). We can play the "Simon Says" game where he is to order us around the room (command speech). He can tell us about what his peers or family do that make him mad or afraid (emotional utterance). By asking him if he had three wishes what he would wish for we can observe his speech in the formulation of thought.

These types of communication and others will help us not only to more fully evaluate the child's speech but to design our therapy. For example if there is a certain type of communication that gives him a lot of trouble we can plan a desensitization program to help him with it. During every session we will try to have him use that type of speech that causes the increase in disfluencies even though we may spend only a short time with it each day. Of course in this desensitization we don't want him to feel too much frustration. If he begins breaking down and stuttering increases we can change and have him use the kind of communication in which he has little trouble. Gradually we can condition him so that he can also master the type of speaking that formerly was difficult.

Some may feel that we are spending too much time in evaluation. We don't agree. If we can locate more of these beginning stutterers and treat them before they develop advanced symptoms our jobs will be easier and more successful.

We will also need to observe the child reacting to communicative stress. By simply pretending not to understand the child as much stress as you wish can be programmed into the situation. The encounter might go something like this:

(C) "Let's pretend that I don't know anything about baseball. It will be your job to teach me."

(S) "What do you want to know about it?"

(C) "Tell me about the batter."

(S) "Well he stands up to the plate and . . ."

(C) "You mean there's a plate like when you eat supper?"

(S) "No, no it's home plate. It's a base."

(C) "Well, what's a base?"

(S) "It's a thing you stand on to be safe."

(C) "Oh, I see, you go up to home and stand on it?"

(S) "No, you stand beside it with a bat."

(C) "What's a bat?"

(S) "It's made of wood."

(C) "Oh, like a tennis racket."

(S) "No, no it's round."

(C) "Well a tennis racket is round."

(S) "But it's long like a stick."

Such a confrontation would be difficult for any child and most of them will soon become frustrated by such demands but what we are interested in studying are the types of disfluencies that arise under this stress. Do they change? Do we see struggle and tension that we hadn't noticed before? Or does the frequency of disfluency but not the severity increase? If this is the case, the child may not be a stutterer. A word of caution. We must of course be careful that we do not overstress the child or spoil our relationship for some children are very easily frustrated and have little tolerance for failure. We must be alert to both their body language and their voice quality as well as their fluency but a good clinician tries to be continually alert to any changes in the feelings of her client and will know when to quit.

Role playing provides another good way of manufacturing communicative stress. Children like role playing. For example, we might play the role of an impatient McDonald's waiter wanting our client to order quickly, or that of a gruff principal or policeman. And we can switch roles too. There are many ways to put communicative pressure on the child. Our intentions are honorable and we never let a child get too frustrated. The important thing is that somehow we get the necessary information. Once we have an idea of his speech under pressure there is no need to continue our stress interviews although later on in therapy we can use similar activities to help us desensitize the child to the communicative stresses to which he is vulnerable.

Direct Confrontation As a Diagnostic Aid

Sometimes in making our diagnosis we confront the child directly: "I'm the speech teacher here at school and I help children who sometimes have trouble talking. How about you? Do you ever have trouble talking?" When doing this it is good to show the child examples of an articulation error, a language error and some mild stuttering samples. In showing him the mild samples we might say:

(C) "All right, how about one like *thi-thi-this*. Ever have one like that? It's kind of like a *bou-bou-bouncing* ball. Do you have any that sound like that?"

(S) "Yeah, sometimes I make a word like that."

Surprisingly often you will get the answer, "Yeah, I stutter when I talk." This however doesn't mean that the child is really a stutterer. He may simply have had some normal disfluencies that someone had once criticized. But in any case we must explore further. (If we find he has been overcriticized we need to help both the child and his parents understand that this is not abnormal behavior and should disappear with time.) We might show him some simple repetitions, prolongations and airflow blockages and ask if he ever does anything that sounds like that. Or we might say, "OK Johnny, I'm going to stutter on some words and you tell me if you have ever said a word like that?" We then show him some samples of stuttering that increase in severity. Even if the child is a real stutterer he will see that he is not as bad as the severe samples would indicate and if he isn't, he will tell you.

After seeing such a child for several sessions and talking with his parents and teacher we should have a fair picture of both his overt and the hidden portion of the child's disfluency problem. If we have a fairly well adjusted child with only some mild disfluencies we probably would not enroll him for therapy.

These then are some of the techniques you can use in obtaining a more reliable differential diagnosis. The important thing is not the activities themselves but the rationale behind them. They are all designed to help us gather information about the disfluent child sitting beside us. Our goal is to determine with some efficiency whether to enroll the child for therapy. Since we are all forced to make these decisions too quickly and with too little knowledge of the child we must continually check for errors in our judgment particularly when we have decided not to enroll a child. Often we have kept in touch with the child's teacher throughout the year in order to check on the child's fluency. Also if you have an unexpected free period take a

23

few minutes to see that child or call his mother. The more we can do to insure the validity of our diagnosis the better. This extra caution will be rewarded in the long run for early detection of stuttering makes for a brighter prognosis.

Indirect Therapy for the Borderline Stutterer

First of all we are going to talk about the stuttering child who has little or no struggle or tension and who has neither shame, guilt nor embarrassment associated with his disfluencies. His only problem seems to be that he has too many of these fluency errors. He would be the mildest stutterer we would accept for therapy, and he is the child that most speech clinicians never work with. Clinicians often say, "Well you know he is so young and has such mild stuttering. Perhaps if we wait a year or two he will outgrow it." We don't feel we should wait. Not only are these mild, borderline stutterers a real joy to work with but their stuttering responds quickly if you can get it soon enough. We must prevent its growth, not ignore it. If we avoid working with these borderline stutterers they will often come back to us in later years, severely handicapped and with much greater needs that require more difficult therapy. Let's get them early!

Once you accept one of these borderline stutterers for therapy the important thing to remember is to keep the sessions casual and indirect. If you do, there is little chance of making the child worse. If he is a kindergartner or even younger it usually means that you will need to get out your toys and let the child play during most of the session, with all communication revolving about the play. During this play activity you will learn many things about the child by seeing how he functions in his own world. Most children when talking directly to adults use a conforming kind of communication and behavior which does not appear in their commentary when playing. Their speech to adults is often artificial and contrived, even stilted but in play the child feels confident and free and he tends to speak that way. The world of play is his world. He will talk to himself and to you in connected phrases rather than offer the usual single-word responses to your questions. All that many of these disfluent children need is a bath of this communicative freedom to heal themselves.

One of the problems of itinerant teachers is that we cannot carry all the toys we might like to use unless we have a bus but it is wise at least to carry a few books for different ages, some farm or zoo animals and some little cars and trucks. All public school clinicians have carrying bags full of interesting junk but the toys selected should be those that evoke speech.

How might we start working with this borderline stutterer, the one who is at a lower rung on the severity continuum? Let us now consider some of the things that might happen in that first session.

(C) "Well Hi Johnny, remember me? I'm the person who came to talk with you the other day. (The child nods his head in recognition.) Today we are going to look at some things in my suitcase. It's this one here." (The clinician then puts the briefcase on the floor or table.)

If we use a table then we need to be careful about our selection of the chairs. It is better to give the child the bigger chair as we take a small one, if the two sizes are available. This puts him in a better position to handle things on the table and it keeps us from being above him. It is good for a child to have his eyes on an equal level with ours. Too often they are forced to look up at us. We have often wondered why more children don't grow up with a permanent crook in their necks.

(C) "Do you know how to open it? (The child begins to push the buttons, trying to open the briefcase. At times we may need to help him but we don't de it for him. We want him to feel some sense of accomplishment immediately.) Good! You figured it out! I have to help some of the other kids do it, older ones than you too! Now look in there and see what you would like to play with today."

(S) "Hey, what are these? Can I look at these?"

(C) "OK. Let's see, what do you want?" (The child dumps the bag of animals and cars on the table.)

(S) "I've got a car like this *wa-wa-one* at home."

(C) "You've got one like that green one at home?"

(S) "*And-And-And* look here's a *lllion.*"

(C) "That's right, a lion. What else have we got here? (The clinician touches some of the toys.) What about this one?"

(S) "*A-A-A* tiger."

(C) "A tiger. That's right." (The child will then often start naming many of the animals.)

In this simple interchange we are trying to do several things at once. We want to convey our warmth and genuine interest and to begin to establish the permissive bond that is so important with the beginning stutterer. The clinician's tone at this time is casual, warm and relaxed, seeking to create an atmosphere of calmness. Because we wish to let the child have as much freedom as possible, we let him set the course of the session. He can choose what and how he wants to play. We are there just to keep the activity within certain limits. We are trying to make talking pleasant while at the same time providing him good speech models. Therefore try to speak simply and slowly but naturally, for we know that if our speech models are too advanced they will have little impact. Occasionally it is wise to insert little repetitions or other mild fluency errors into our own speech. This, of course, doesn't mean that the clinician should talk like a child for they will immediately recognize the fraudulence. No, we always talk like the adults we are but we can talk a bit more simply and without hurry. The session continues:

> (S) "Oh, look here's an *a-a-a-alligator.*"
> (C) "That's right an *a-alligator.* Where does he live?"
> (S) *"By-By-By* the water."
> (C) "That's right he likes to be by the water just like we do."

It is important that the clinician at times echoes back some of the child's speech as well as presenting better models. This does many positive things. It shows him that you have received his message, that you are interested in what he is saying, and that you are not concerned about any stuttering he might have had. This doesn't mean that you should parrot mechanically everything the child says. That would be foolish and the child would soon catch on. Instead we try to reflect in our own words the basic idea of what the child is saying just as we often do in talking to our adult friends. How often we hear this same type of exchange in our everyday life. "I saw a good movie last night." "You saw a movie?" "Yeah, we saw Star Wars." "Star Wars, I've heard about it. Is it as good as they say?" "It was crazy." "Really crazy huh?" etc. etc. This reflecting is just a friendly way of talking with one another. Another benefit of this form of echo talking or reflecting is that it encourages the child to talk further. Not only will the child be talking willingly but usually he will be leading the conversation. This is much better than having him continually answering our questions. Any child is much freer and more spontaneous when he doesn't have to endure a cross examination. Most questions involve too much demand. We use them sparingly.

Modeling Milder Forms of Stuttering

In this echo speaking or reflecting we occasionally provide the child with a better model of stuttering than the kind he shows. If possible we want to erase the memory of the abnormality of his stuttered words. When a child says *"a-a-a-alligator"*, some trace of that disfluency is being recorded in his brain and we should try to reduce the impact of that recording. If he hears us say it fluently or less abnormally soon after he has stuttered, it should help to minimize some of the ill effects of that particular moment of stuttering. Thus, the child is being corrected without his being aware of it and in fact the interchange seems pleasant to him. How different this is from the kind of correction that he gets from his parents and classmates. Most little stuttering children fear and hate the constant correction that they must endure. Say it again! Say it again! Slow down! Don't stutter!

Moreover, when most people correct a stuttering child, they merely demand that he say the word as they do, completely fluently. Sometimes he just can't and then he tends to become aware of his trouble. Instead, we might use a mild and easy repetition or two on one of the words on which he has stuttered much more severely. The reason for this procedure is that we should immediately begin to provide models of less abnormal stuttering. Stuttering can reverse its course and it is vitally important that the child learns early that there is no need to force or struggle. We are not asking him or attempting to teach him to be entirely fluent immediately. We know this is unreasonable. Instead, our basic goal is to make the stuttering milder for we have found, over and over again, that once the stuttering begins to get less severe, it will eventually disappear.

Reducing the severity of a stuttered word is more important than reducing the frequency of stuttering. One moment of severe stuttering can be much more traumatic than many little disfluencies. If the child feels "stuck" and unable to move forward, how quickly the emotions of fear, helplessness, and embarrassment can overwhelm him. We must do all we can to reduce these moments of severity so that those negative feelings do not get a chance to grow. If we reduce the severity we also reduce the emotions of fear and frustration that breed more stuttering. Let us break the vicious circle as soon as possible and reverse it.

What we are doing then is to show the borderline stutterer a better way of responding to the interruptions in his speech by modeling our own casual acceptance of our mild disfluencies. We show him that we can put them into our own mouth without getting upset. We don't overdo this of course. Often, in a session, we might insert some mild stutterings into our own speech only once or twice and, of course, at other times it is wise just to say his stuttered word fluently. We keep it natural!

The Compulsive Talker

Another reason for reflecting the child's speech is that it keeps him from running away with the conversation. We have seen children who once they began talking would not stop, compulsively piling up one moment of stuttering after another into a torrent of broken speech. There are many possible explanations for this compulsivity. Possibly the child has a real fear of being interrupted and so he tries to keep talking for as long as possible. Perhaps he uses his constant verbalization as a strategy for dominating those around him, in particular the speech teacher. Or it may be due to the fear of having trouble starting again or to convince himself that he really can be fluent. For most of these children starting a sentence is where his stuttering most often occurs and so they speak without period or pause. This compulsive speech as a reaction to disfluency is dangerous. By reflecting what he has just said, we can break it up without frustrating him.

Again there are other children who because of communicative deprivation at home or at school just hunger for a chance to talk and the clinician may be the only one they can talk to. Such a child often comes from a family with older brothers and sisters who rarely let him get a word in edgewise or who constantly interrupt or correct him. With these speech-hungry children we give them as much opportunity to talk as possible but even with these children we can use this reflecting kind of speech to help guide the conversation, to show that we are listening and to provide better models of easier stuttering and normal speech.

Often when a stuttering child is also a compulsively fast talker, we ask him to dictate. He soon realizes that we cannot write fast enough so this helps him slow down. Such an activity also provides a good opportunity for repeating back the child's speech to him since we must continually tell him what we have written. Children love this dictating to adults. It makes them feel important.

The Ongoing Diagnosis

During the first few sessions this reflecting may be the only outward thing you do. However, indirectly it creates an opportunity for making the observations you need to understand the child and to establish the kind of warm relationship required for all good therapy. In these observations we should be looking for many things, both emotional and physical. We will not attempt to cover all of them since each clinician has her own set of questions concerning the children she sees but some to consider are: (1) How strong is his self concept? (2) How does he view his role in the family? (3) How does he relate to other children? (4) Is he aggressive or withdrawn? (5) Is he determined to talk in spite of his stuttering? (6) How aware does he seem to be of his stuttering? (7) Does he ever try to avoid or substitute a non-feared word? (8) Does he ever try to cover his mouth when he stutters? (9) Does he ever use a timing gesture to help get a word out? (10) Are there some sounds or words that continually seem to give him trouble? (11) Is his stuttering usually on the first word of utterances? (12) Does his stuttering usually occur on the first sound or syllable? (13) How much fear and embarrassment does he feel when talking? And there are many more.

At this time it is important to make a tape recording of the child because you will use it later to practice the child's kind of stuttering and his overall speech patterns. We need to be able to imitate the child's stuttering with fidelity. Many clinicians fail to do this although it is probably the best way to understand not only stuttering in general but also an individual child's particular difficulty. There seems to be a special kind of empathic understanding that comes when we feel his stuttering in our own mouth. It's what happens to actors when they put on the costume after memorizing the script and for a brief time seem to become the character they are portraying. One cannot understand the stuttering child nor help him find better ways of talking without actually feeling first hand the stuttering he experiences. Besides, we will need the tape recording later on to assess his improvement.

Initiating a More Direct Approach

When should we become more direct in our confrontation of the child's stuttering? There are some indications to scrutinize before deciding on a more direct approach. Is he comfortable in your presence? Has he begun to accept and trust you? At times these questions can be answered positively even during the first session but for most children it takes longer. When he does show us that he is comfortable we can begin casually and calmly to confront the stuttering itself, but generally let us be willing to wait. The clinical relationship should never be forced. We move in and touch the stuttering and then move out again, back to our play, then back to confronting it. This excerpt may illustrate how we might do so.

(C) "Now I'm going to take this *re-re-rred* car. Hey, I got stuck on that didn't I? Let me try it again. It's a *re-rred* car. There that was easier but let me try it again once more. It's a *rred* car. That's better. I kind of bounced on it the first time." (The clinician then returns to the play activity.)

In this little episode the confrontation process has begun. The child has been shown that he is not the only one who can stutter occasionally, that there is at least one adult who can unemotionally stop, describe what happened, correct it and go on. No sweat! No big thing! The casualness with which the comments were made was more important than the words. If the child is really stuttering he will be relieved to have it come out in the open and he will then be able to give you more of his trust.

Another byproduct of the clinician's simulation of moments of stuttering is that it gives her an opportunity to observe the stutterer's reaction. Some children's eyes widen dramatically when we do this for the first time; others may laugh nervously. Some may tell you that you stuttered just like they do. Others will even try to help by saying the word for you when you try it again. Such reactions can give us a good clue as to how he feels about his stuttering. (Incidentally, most of the children know what they do is "stuttering", no matter how carefully others have avoided using the label. This is true even for those whose parents claim that the child doesn't have any awareness of his stuttering! The child knows! Let's not pretend that there's nothing wrong with his fluency if he is really having trouble.)

Out of such little confrontations the foundation for future exploration of the child's stuttering has been poured. It sometimes even happens that a child may want some immediate information about stuttering and will ask you directly if you stutter too. If he does, you might say calmly, "Well yes, I sometimes bounce on a word like *thi-thi-this* just like you did a little while ago. Most people do and some do it more often than others. You sometimes seem to have more than most kids." Occasionally a child will then tell you that there are times when he stutters or repeats and that his Mom and Dad get mad at him for it and can you help him stop doing it? To such a direct question you might reply, "I see lots of kids everyday who repeat or get stuck on their words or who stutter. As the speech teacher my job is to help kids learn to talk better." This seems logical to the child and he is left feeling more secure. Of course you should attempt at a later date to go back and get more information from him about his parent's reactions to his stuttering but for now we have probably done enough and it is time to play and talk again.

Another important result of such a confrontation episode is that it gives you some indication of how fast you should proceed in therapy. The child's reaction may tell you to move very cautiously or, on the contrary, to push on ahead. By taking advantage of these little encounters and recognizing the implications of the signals the child gives you should reduce your worry about making the stuttering worse. This should not be new to you. You are already doing this same assessment in your articulation therapy. We are always evaluating how much a child can handle before becoming overloaded.

If the child seems to be embarrassed or upset by your pseudo-stuttering then you will know that you must go very slowly and work hard to develop more trust and acceptance. Nevertheless you should continue on occasion to insert some mild stuttering in your speech without commenting on it. He'll get used to it if you do so calmly and casually. Eventually there will come a time when he will not respond emotionally. When the child is able to react to our stuttering with little concern, then we can move forward. After all, one of the goals with all stutterers is to reduce the emotionality surrounding the disorder. For young children this approach seems to be most suitable.

One of our colleagues told of having a difficult time putting this mild, pseudo-stuttering into her own speech. It had always made her feel uncomfortable and somehow fraudulent. One day however while using a hand puppet she made a discovery. She could make "Charley" the puppet stutter! Soon she learned how to move "Charley's" mouth so that it looked like stuttering. Her little stuttering client was so fascinated by "Charley" that she was successfully able to use the puppet not only for desensitization purposes but also to help demonstrate a milder form of stuttering.

After he has become familiar with our occasional mild stutterings we then try to get him more actively involved in our demonstrations. We might proceed as follows:

(C) "I'm going to drive *my-my-mmmy* . . . Oops! There I did it again. Did you hear that?"

(S) "Yes, you stuttered a little."

(C) "On what?"

(S) "You stuttered on *my.*"

(C) "I said that word *my* kind of funny didn't it? I think it sounded like this, *my-my-mmmy,* didn't it? It's like bouncing a ball
isn't it?" (The clinician pretends to be bouncing a ball as she
stutters on the word *ball.*) "Do you ever have words come out
like that, like the *bou-bou-bouncing ball*? Or hang on to a
sound like *mmmmmmy* on the word *my*?"

(S) "Yes I do it sometimes. My mom says it's because I try to talk
too fast."

Most stutterers no matter how young they are will usually admit
having this type of easy stuttering and when they do the door to the
child's problem his been opened. Dealing with the stuttering in this
relaxed but straightforward manner may seem too direct an approach
for some clinicians. They may feel that all confrontation should
be avoided since it will only confirm in the child's mind that
he is a "stutterer". We have not found this to be true. Children
usually breathe a sigh of relief, when at last someone is willing to talk
to them about their stuttering. This careful confrontation just makes
it easier for them to objectify their stuttering as a problem not a
mysterious curse.

Once again, we don't pursue the matter too strongly. It is enough
that the ice has been broken and the impact made. A seemingly
insignificant event has cleared a path for future advances in therapy.

As we have said, most children, even the young ones, already refer
to their disfluencies as stuttering, sometimes even to disfluencies
which are not. Although we should not flinch from their use of the
word stuttering, this label, of course does little to objectively
describe the behavior. To many children the word stuttering is a term
colored by emotionality and threat and so we therefore prefer to talk
about the child's disfluencies in terms of what actually is happening.
If he is repeating, then let's refer to it as bouncing because that is
what it sounds like and the children understand what bouncing
means. If he is prolonging then we refer to it as stretching out a
sound or holding onto a sound. If the child is blocking the airflow,
then we refer to it as being stuck. These are fairly objective terms
that the child understands and so when we use them we are doing
much to lessen the emotional stigma that surrounds stuttering. Let's
talk about what he does.

Should the clinician only use the words disfluency or nonfluency
with stuttering children? To most children these terms are meaning-
less. They are not in his vocabulary. Moreover they have no more
objectivity than the word stuttering. If you use them you run some

risk that the child will suspect you of trying to cover up his problem, that you too are flinching from its confrontation. He doesn't want you to protect him; he wants you to help him! Many other adults in his life have beaten around the verbal bush using such terms as hesitation, speech problem, fluency problem or "It". To him "non-fluency" or "disfluency" are cop-out words. The child has that sick feeling that the real word, the right word is *stuttering* and that it is so awful that people don't even dare mention it. Every child in the "bluebird" reading group knows well that being a "bluebird" means that he is a poor reader.

Now let us return for a moment to our previous encounter and see what might happen if the child had responded like this:

(C) "Do you ever make words come out like that, like the *bou-bou-bouncing ball*?"

(S) "No, my baby brother does sometimes but I never stutter." (This reaction is unusual but if there is one thing that we learn from stutterers it is to expect the unexpected. An appropriate response to his denial might sound like this:)

(C) "So your baby brother sometimes bounces on his words. So do I and so do most people sometimes."

Nothing is accomplished by arguing with the child. Just go along with him acceptingly. He either is really not aware of his disfluencies or else (which is probably more often the case) he is ashamed and not yet ready to admit having them. And even if he does not actually have a younger sibling who stutters we can ask him to tell us how he sounds when he does stutter and what his mom and dad tell this real or imaginary brother to do about it. However it may be wise to point out calmly one of his own repetitions to him soon after this complete denial. If he is ever to trust us he must recognize that we are honest. For example as we return to our verbal and nonverbal play, he might say:

(S) "Give me the *ti-ti-tiger*."

(C) "Seems to me I just heard you bounce on the word *tiger*. Didn't you say *ti-ti-tiger*? Sometimes you bounce on your words *ju-just* like I do."

(S) "Yeah, sometimes I do but not very much." (We then go back to our play.)

And so even in the case of the child who denies his stuttering the confrontation has been accomplished in a casual, nonthreatening way. We will now be able to talk descriptively about the child's speech behaviors feeling sure that he knows what we are talking about. Moreover, we can hope now that he is also beginning to understand that with us stuttering is not evil, not unmentionable, that it carries no threat.

Strengthening the Fluency

Another goal for these borderline stutterers is to show them how fluent they are most of the time. Why should we dwell only on just the child's stuttering? He also has substantial amounts of fluency and surely we should try to reinforce that. If we have been able to help relieve the child's fear and shame and can make the fluency strong enough it will tend eventually to overwhelm the stuttering. But how do we encourage a child's fluency without making him feel that fluency is good and disfluency is bad? Our answer is that it is quite possible to reinforce fluency strongly without praising it or condemning stuttering.

First we must make the child aware of his fluency. In much the same way that we focused some attention on his disfluencies we now want to focus on his fluency. For example, we might do something like this:

(C) "OK, now let's do some work. Let me have all the toys over here." (The clinician gathers all the toys in a pile beside her.) "Now see if you can say just what I say. The car is red."

(S) "It's red."

(C) "That's not what I said. Listen again. The car is red. Can you say that?"

(S) "The car is red."

(C) "That's right. The car is red. Did you bounce on any of those words?"

(S) "No." (The clinician puts the red car over beside the child.)

(C) "Now say this; 'The kangaroo has a long tail'."

(S) "The kangaroo has a long tail."

(C) "Say it again but put your hand over your mouth so you can *feel* how you said it. Feel your lips moving, and your jaw and tongue." (The child does so and the clinician puts the kangaroo over beside him.) "Now how about this one? Say: 'The elephant has a trunk', but this time shut your eyes and listen to how you say it."

(S) "*Th-th-the* elephant has a trunk."

(C) "Did you bounce on any of those words?"

(S) "Yeah. I said *th-th-the*."

(C) "Yes, I thought I heard you say *th-th-the elephant* too. If you say it without bouncing, how would it sound?"

(S) "The elephant has a trunk."

(C) "Yes. That probably felt and sounded smoother."

After several of these interchanges most children are usually able to accurately assess their own fluency, and of course the child's pile of toys always grows far bigger than the clinician's. We can always schedule our mild penalties, withholdings and rewards so the child is going to succeed more than he fails.

Another similar game is one called, "Catch Me". First we will give him a phrase to repeat after us, then have him give us one. It is the child's job to catch the clinician when she shows some disfluency. Children love this for nothing is more delightful for a child than to be able to correct an adult.

The game might proceed something like this:

(C) "Now this time we are both going to take turns talking." (The clinician sweeps up all the toys and puts them in a pile beside her.) "Now tell me something about the elephant."

(S) "The elephant has a trunk."

(C) "Did you bounce on any of the words?"

(S) "No." (The clinician puts the elephant over beside the child.)

(C) "Now it's my turn. This kangaroo has big feet. Did I bounce on any of those words?"

(S) "No." (The clinician puts the kangaroo next to her.)

(C) "How about this one?"

(S) "The alligator has sharp teeth."

(C) "No bounces there. My turn. The car *i-i-is green*. Did I have any bounces?"

(S) "No."

(C) "Oh, I sure fooled you that time. I went the car *i-i-is green* and you didn't catch me." (The clinician puts the car on her own pile. The child says another fluent sentence and it is the clinician's turn again.) "The giraffe has a *bi-bi-big neck.*"

(S) "Hey you stuttered on that."

(C) "What word did I bounce on?"

(S) "You bounced on *big neck.*"

(C) "That's right you caught me that time. You get to have the giraffe in your pile." (The child is laughing with glee at this point.)

(S) "Hey you know what? I've got more than you now."

(C) "Well how many do you have?" (The child counts proudly and they continue.)

(S) "The lion has *a-a-a* long tail."

(C) "I caught you that time. You went the lion has *a-a-a* long tail. I heard you bounce on that. So I get the lion in my pile."

Now let us provide a word of caution about the pseudo-stuttering that the clinician uses in these desensitization encounters. First of all she should try to keep out the use of the schwa vowel "uh" when repeating a syllable. For instance, make sure that in your repetitions you say *reh-reh-red car* rather than *ruh-ruh-red*. At first this may take some conscious effort since the schwa vowel tends to creep in. Also make sure that the repetitions are evenly paced and tension free. You should not be demonstrating stuttering with struggle but rather an easier relaxed form of stuttering. We must create models of easier stuttering not more severe ones.

The above activities may have helped us in several ways; (1) We have concretely demonstrated to the child that he has good fluency and that he can feel it. (2) He has confronted his stuttering with a clinician who is both understanding and forgiving. (3) The emotionality of stuttering has been reduced through our fun activities. (4) And he has had a chance to get back at the world by being able to correct an adult who occasionally pretends to stutter.

We not only want children to speak fluently we also want them to experience the feel of fluency through their senses. We have had children talk while having their fingers over their lips so that they can better feel their lips moving fluently. Resting their chin on their hand helps them feel the jaw movements. A magnifying mirror aimed at their lips will give them visual feedback of fluency. Clinicians have been leery of such an activity because they wonder what happens if the child should stutter and is forced to see his magnified lips jammed up on a sound. This happens rarely because the visual feedback seems to promote fluency but if it did we should treat it with casual curiosity asking the child to describe what he saw. We may have him imitate the moment of stuttering again so that we can study it and objectify the experience thus removing much of the fear and mystery which surrounds stuttering. Take the mirror yourself and imitate his stuttering and both of you can examine your lips and describe what is happening.

Others have used a cardboard sheet and cut out two eyeholes and a big hole for the mouth. The child holds this up to his face and looks into a mirror. His vision is focused onto his mouth thus making use of the visual feedback.

Another easy way of reinforcing a child's fluency is to let him monopolize verbally the session when he is having a good speech day. Early in the session we try to assess the child's fluency, for his speech may vary a great deal from day to day. We have seen children enter a session on Monday in a bad mood and stuttering quite frequently and then on Tuesday come in happy and with no observable stuttering. We use these mood swings to our advantage. Often a child will come in happy and speaking fluently. All is well with his world. During these times we encourage him to speak as much as he can, letting him flood his system with fluency. Fluency seems to breed more fluency. Usually the child doesn't need much encouragement. He wants to talk. In any case it is our job on these good days to get out of the way and let him go.

If, however, the child is having much trouble on a certain day we use a lot of nonverbal activities. Perhaps we spend the time on the floor playing with toys while keeping the session unstructured and relaxed. We may play a game that he enjoys, one which doesn't require any complicated speech. For twenty minutes we try to bring some pleasantness into his life. Possibly this brief oasis will be enough to change his whole day. All of us have bad days and it's good when someone shows us some extra kindness or thoughtfulness during such a time. Although we usually keep the majority of our sessions unstructured we often try to spend at least five minutes on some fluency producing exercise. Even on his bad days we want him to experience some fluency and so may provide even more opportunity when he is having difficulty.

Of course much of the time he will be on some middle ground, neither very fluent or disfluent. Only occasionally have we seen children who might change radically during a session and realize that he's stuttering a lot more, or that he has stopped stuttering completely. If these mid-session changes occur we adjust accordingly.

Unfortunately too many of us ignore or don't recognize these signs of change and continue with our original therapy plans. By being alert to the child's condition when he enters our room, we can better meet his current needs.

Prosody and rhythm are often not adequately developed in these young disfluent children. So we may have them tap out syllables on the table as they make up phrases. Once they get the idea they become very fluent and their prosody improves. It may sound mechanical at first but they soon learn to tap the proper rhythm. With some however you will need to talk and tap in unison until they get the idea. Some have accused us of teaching "tricks" and using the hackneyed methods of the old "stuttering institutes". But we are not teaching them tricks or bad habits. The tapping out of syllables may last for only five minutes during a session. We are not teaching the tapping as a method to maintain fluency but rather to help a child feel the prosody and rhythm of speech. In the unlikely event that a child did start to tap out all of his words we could quickly phase out the activity by having him vary the tapping and then to simply have him imagine he was tapping. Tapping is burdensome and no child wants extra labor when speaking.

As we become familiar with our client we learn the types of speaking activities that he can do fluently. The descriptive type of speech will often yield good fluency. Children find it easy to talk about a picture or go through a familiar book telling us a story from the pictures. Having the pictures to look at helps the child in the formulation of language. For example we can give the child one point everytime he says a phrase fluently and we get a point whenever he stutters on a word. Always his point total will be much larger than ours. When he begins to have 90% fluency in this activity we can then program some mild fluency disruptors in order to desensitize him to them. Turning our back to the child will often cause some mild stuttering but first we tell him that we are trying to make it harder for him to talk. As he becomes accustomed to this challenge we may get up and look out the window as he says his phrases. Once again we tell him that we are trying to trick him, to make it harder for him so that we can score some points. Or we may talk at the same time he is talking or try to interrupt him. We have used a little transistor radio and told him to make up phrases while it is playing. Or, while saying a phrase in unison, we may do some pseudo-stuttering on one of the words, asking him to resist us and not to let us make him stutter.

We have also used role playing effectively in this desensitization to fluency disruption. In the fall during our diagnostic exam we used the technique to assess his problem but now we try to condition him to remain fluent while playing these roles. We might play an impatient waitress or a gruff policeman or principal and it is his job to resist us and to keep talking fluently. At first we will make it quite easy for him to succeed; later we will apply more pressure. We always try to program only enough pressure so that he will succeed more than he breaks down. We build on success rather than failure. The more he succeeds the harder we pressure him but make sure he always wins in the end.

Many times we leave the therapy room for these desensitization activities. Talking while walking is sometimes more difficult for some children. In an empty gym we may stand on opposite sides of the room while he is making up phrases. (It is often harder for the stutterer to talk when his listener is far away.) We may explore what happens when he gets up on stage. Perhaps the child can pretend to give a brief report to an imaginary audience. Or we have gone out on the playground where we need to shout to each other. Throughout all of these activities we are giving him points or some acknowledgement for remaining fluent while losing points for stuttering but it is all done in the spirit of a game or challenge and we never continue an activity that produces more failure than success. If he is failing to maintain fluency in one activity we try to decrease the stress during the activity so that he can succeed or shift to another. We keep the encounter fun and rewarding although often we may give him a taste of failure so he knows we aren't babying him. We want him to feel challenged and under some threat of failure for otherwise the activities have little value.

We need to find ways for showing the child how fluent he is most of the time. Too many of these children think only about their stuttering. The only words they remember are those they stutter upon. We want them to shift their attention to their abundant fluency. We need to increase the amount of the child's fluency while at the same time helping him build up a tolerance for and a defense against those fluency disruptors that face him everyday. If we can design our therapy to accomplish these goals we will not need to worry much about the child's occasional mild disfluencies.

Often with these mild stuttering children the fluency training consumes the major portion of our therapy time. There is little need of working continually on only the stuttering when in reality very little stuttering remains. Nevertheless we do not neglect the stuttering entirely. Every child needs some basic information about stuttering and we give it to him even though we spend most of our time increasing and strengthening the child's fluency. He needs to know that he is not alone in his stuttering and that we understand and are not afraid of it. He needs some understanding of what stuttering is and why it is happening to him. This understanding will help to remove any of the mystery that often surrounds his stuttering. If he has received any emotional hurts because of his stuttering these will need our empathetic understanding. So we do not believe that it is wise to work entirely or solely on either the fluency or the stuttering. We devote time to each one appropriately.

Conclusion

These then are the kinds of things we might do with the child whom we can perhaps call a borderline stutterer. Our therapy time is used primarily to get us acquainted with him and his possible stuttering. We want to make sure that he is not hiding any real stuttering. We help him become more fluent. We provide models. Our sessions are casual, indirect and nonthreatening. We provide an opportunity for free, pleasant communication. Once we feel reasonably certain that the child is just going through a period of disfluency we can dismiss him from our caseload.

Some may criticize us for having been either overcautious or overzealous. Many of these children would have become normally fluent without our intervention. However, we feel that we have invested our time wisely. First of all we have shown that teacher who referred him that we appreciate her concerns and are responding to them. Secondly, we have had a chance to deal with any of the fears and questions that the parents may have. Thirdly, we have become familiar with the child so that if he does at any time have some real stuttering we can step into the situation with a better start. Fourthly, if the child is a real stutterer who can hide his stuttering we will be able to diagnose it during this period of observation and put him on our regular therapy schedule. On the other hand were his stuttering left untreated for a year or two then we would probably have a more serious problem on our hands in the future. Finally, both the clinician and the child have benefited from the time together. If the communicative sessions are interesting, casual and relaxed any child will benefit from this extra attention and stimulation. This kind of therapy could be used with every child in a classroom and all of them would communicate better.

The clinician will also gain personal benefit from these sessions. She will learn something of what beginning stuttering looks like in all its variations and will become more familiar with the range of normal disfluencies. This will help overcome her fears of working with stutterers because these children are so mild she will not be threatened. They have not been hurt or damaged by society as has the advanced stutterer. They are free spirits and truly joys to work with.

The Mild Stutterer

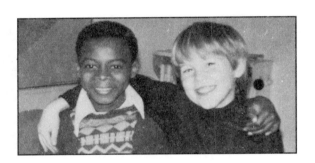

The Mild Stutterer

Description of the Mild Stutterer as Distinguished from the Borderline Stutterer

Now let us move along the continuum to the child who is showing signs of more advanced stuttering. He may show some struggle or tension when speaking. He might be using the schwa vowel in his repetitions or they may be uneven or forced or be accompanied by a pitch rise. As he attempts certain words the airflow may occasionally be blocked. He might even show some of the secondary danger signals such as shyness or nervousness when speaking. Any one of these danger signs or a combination of them tends to indicate that this particular child may be beginning to stutter more severely.

This picture is quite different from that shown by the children we have previously discussed. Although still fairly mild, these children definitely stutter. Unfortunately they too are not worked with by public school clinicians. Although they recognize that the child is stuttering, since the disorder is still mild, they are afraid that any therapy might make him worse. Besides they always have the hope that he may outgrow it on his own. Their caseloads are already full and it is often difficult to find a place for such a child on their schedule. There are always reasons, good reasons, but if we are really honest with ourselves we must admit that our fear of making him worse and our own feelings of inadequacy are the major reasons for telling the parents and teacher that he will probably outgrow it in time. But usually this mild stutterer can benefit from our help and should get it. If we keep in mind the casual and relaxed sessions described in connection with the borderline stutterer then there is no reason to expect that this child will get worse if a similar approach is used.

We must realize that stuttering is a progressive disorder, and that an occasional child may get worse despite our efforts. This however should not imply that we have been at fault. There are many forces in the school, home or playground over which we may have little control that can worsen the stuttering. While it is possible that some of these children may attain normal fluency without your help, it is also possible (even probable) that they are in danger of becoming confirmed severe stutterers. All we can say is that when a child is in danger, the clinician should step in and not wash her hands of the responsibility.

Many of the therapy activities we used with the borderline stutterer can also be used with the mild stutterer. We don't suddenly use a new set of techniques simply because we have a more advanced stutterer on our hands. What changes is the directness of the approach. Once again we should keep the sessions warm and friendly. We want to provide a permissive communicative atmosphere in which the child can feel free to talk despite any stuttering that may occur.

The Outline of Treatment: Gradual but Direct Confrontation

The basic aim of treatment is to prevent the child from reacting to the stuttering experience by avoidance or struggle. The clinician must understand how traumatic it can be to find yourself repeating interminably, or to find yourself prolonging a sound you have already produced, or to experience the greater trauma of not being able to move your mouth or tongue and being incapable of producing voice. These are frightening experiences for a little child and we've got to take the mystery and fear out of them as soon as possible before he begins to react to them by struggle or avoidance. Most of the handicap of stuttering arises from the child's reactions to these stuttering experiences. If we can make them benign, he'll heal himself.

Some stutterers however show these danger symptoms but apparently do not react to them. Don't let their lack of outward reaction fool you into thinking that no danger exists. We have heard many clinicians say: "Well he is doing some obvious mild stuttering but he doesn't seem to react to it. Besides he's such a happy child." The "happy stutterer", who doesn't seem to react to his stuttering probably falls into one of two categories. He has either learned how to hide his emotions, or he is trying to ignore his stuttering.

Both problems need our help. The children who hide their emotions have an obvious need to talk with someone who will understand. The needs of the "happy stutterer", on the other hand are not so obvious but we must recognize that this child is walking a narrow path. Society is cruel to all who stray from the norm. Sooner or later he will feel the pain of being different. How nice it would be if a warm, gentle clinician can help him face his stuttering before others force that recognition traumatically. Shall we leave him defenseless? If a child can learn about stuttering in a happy way, he will not be so vulnerable. He won't have to struggle or avoid or build up the negative emotional reactions that will make his stuttering more severe.

Once again we will be in no rush to confront the child with his disfluencies. Our pace in therapy is relaxed but we must be ready to seize any opportunity the child may give us to discuss the problem calmly. That is why a detailed therapy plan for each session is often counterproductive although this does not mean that we should have no idea of what we plan to accomplish. However the plan should be a general one which will enable us at any moment to make adjustments. Often there may be something we hadn't planned to introduce for several sessions but if the opportunity is there we must take advantage of it. The child must be *ready* for our new ideas and concepts if he is to profit from them. The key here is not only to be ready when the opportunity for a peak experience presents itself but also to guide the sessions so that more of these opportunities have a chance to happen.

The First Confrontation

A good way to begin the confrontation of the child's stuttering is by first using some of our own pseudo-stuttering as an example, and then talking about it. Then we can discuss his stuttering. This approach is much easier for the child. He feels less selfconscious and has more understanding when it is done this way. If we immediately demand that he face his stuttering there is a good chance that he will become too embarrassed, resentful or confused to be able to follow our suggestions.

 (C) "Give me that *re-re-red* . . . Oops. I got stuck on that one. Let me try it again . . . *Re-re-red* car. There that was better.

With a shy child or one whose strength is doubtful this might be all we need do at any one time. In fact we might do it several times over a period of two or three sessions before trying anything further. But with most children you can see by the reaction on their faces that they are interested. In fact some have even volunteered the words, "Hey, you stuttered on that." Or they may say, "Sometimes I stutter on my words like that too." Children who respond in this way are giving us an opportunity to make further progress during the session. And so we would further explore the child's stuttering and his feelings about it. Eventually we would do the same exploration with the shy and withdrawn child. The only difference is that we would greatly slow down the pace of confrontation for the shy child. What you might cover in one or two sessions with one child might take several weeks with another. This of course, is where your skills as a clinician come in. The experienced clinician seems to know when to move ahead and when to hold back. But if you feel that you might have trouble with this don't become alarmed or use your uncertainty as an excuse for not working with the stutterer.

Actually, it is quite easy to judge when you are progressing too rapidly. The child may look away or become restless or he may pretend to ignore you or try to change the subject. Through many signs and signals the child will show you that you are going too fast, are being too direct. We really shouldn't worry too much about making mistakes in pacing our therapy. All of us make them and most children are quick to let us know when we do, so we can slow down until he is ready to move on. This is why it is so important not to be tied down to a strict therapy timetable. We must be able to move fast or slow at a moments notice.

Let us return again to our therapy session:

(C) "I kind of bounced on that word didn't I? It's kind of like *bou-bou-bouncing* a ball. (The clinician bounces an imaginary ball as she makes the repetition.) Do you ever bounce on your words like that?"

(S) "Yeah, sometimes."

(C) "Some kids who come to see me get stuck on their words like this. (The clinician demonstrates blocking the airflow on a word.) Do you ever do that?"

(S) "Sometimes."

(C) "Or sometimes they might hold on to a sound too long like *th----is*. Do you ever make one sound like that?"

(S) "Sometimes."

With most children this is all we may need to do in one session. However some children seem to be able to handle more confrontation and if they can we might continue with some general probing of their emotional responses to their stuttering.

(C) "Does it make you mad when you *bou-bou-bounce* on a word like that?"

(S) "No, but sometimes I try to talk slow and that makes the words come out better."

(C) "Well who told you that talking slower might help?"

(S) "Oh, my dad told me that."

(C) "What other things have your mom and dad told you to help with some of those words?"

(S) "Oh, just to talk slower and to try not to make so many mistakes."

(C) "The trouble is that sometimes it's hard to talk slow, isn't it?

And sometimes even when you do talk slower you still might have trouble with a word. How about the kids in your room, do they ever try to make fun of you when you bounce or get stuck?"

(S) "No . . . Well sometimes *Ji-Ji-Jimmy* Jones does it but my teacher tells him to shut up, because it's not nice to laugh at other kids. Sometimes my sssssssister teases me too and my mom tells her not to do it. Sometimes I punch her right in the stomach."

(C) "So you're pretty tough are you?"

(S) "Yeah, and I punched that Jimmy Jones this morning too."

(C) "So you punched old Jimmy. Is that the kid who sometimes teases you?"

(S) "Yeah, I'm not afraid of him."

We would probably not try to return the subject back to stuttering immediately. We can continue our exploration of his stuttering in our next session. If the flow of his conversation leads us to feel that he really wants to talk further about his stuttering of course we would help him do so. But usually we just let him talk freely. He needs a permissive listener he can trust.

One of the questions that we need answered concerns the child's reaction to his stuttering. Although we cannot accept his reply as the whole truth it may at least begin to answer the question. In the example just cited, the child denied any anger when stuttering although most of the rest that he said indicates some hostility feelings directed elsewhere. The clinician wouldn't interpret these to the child but she would certainly note the context. And she would note that the boy had already begun to react to penalty by aggression.

We have found that although most mild stutterers show little hostility concerning their stuttering, it is not unusual to have a child tell us that his stuttering indeed makes him angry. With these children we would try to empathize with their feelings and give them a chance to vent these hostilities over several therapy sessions. With one of our client's his verbalizing of this hatred of stuttering was the most important single factor in his recovery.

In our example the clinician also gathered some important information about the parent's reactions to the child's stuttering. This information would, of course, not be used to condemn the parents but rather to help us understand the client. In talking with the stutterer we should always be careful not to criticize the suggestions of his parents no matter how unwise they may be. No child should be forced to choose between his parents and his clinician. Instead it is our job to have all of us work together as a team. In the example the clinician didn't criticize the parents but rather she merely tried to show the child she understood that the advice didn't always work, thereby relieving him of any guilt feelings. Some children, because their parents advice has been unsuccessful, feel that they are to blame for not having tried hard enough to follow their parents impossible demands such as "always think before you speak."

In our example you will note that the child also began telling the clinician about the reactions of his classmates and how he dealt with them. This particular child appeared to be able to cope with the reactions of his peers. Although some might disapprove of his coping behavior it appears, at least on the surface, to have satisfied him. We should always be concerned when a child has not learned ways of handling mockery and teasing, for this impotence often begins a vicious circle with evil consequences. The child begins to hide his stuttering and to avoid social contacts. If he retreats into a lonely world of isolation and shame the seeds of severe stuttering will grow quickly in such fertile soil. Therefore instead of feeling a need to condemn him for his aggression we would be relieved to find that he is open and straightforward concerning the reactions of others to his stuttering. This aggression is not at all pathological. In fact it is a perfectly logical and normal way for a six year old boy to handle such a situation. Also the withholding of moral judgment has probably helped the clinician gain the child's acceptance. Adults are forever inflicting moral judgments on their children. How nice to meet one adult who is different, one who understands. During his account of his aggression the child will often scrutinize you carefully for he needs to know if he can trust you. We are not the only ones doing a diagnostic examination in such encounters.

We should realize that much of the time the child will be fantasizing in this free uninhibited talking and that what he tells us may not be the truth. He might be afraid of Jimmy Jones and that punch he told us about was just a mythical one. It doesn't matter. Whatever he tells us helps us know him and his stuttering better and he needs to relieve his tension.In such a monolog we would merely reflect back to him his feelings acceptingly. At the same time, this echoing or reflecting can give us another opportunity to model a better way of stuttering. It also lets him know that we are following him and are interested in his message.

Sooner or later there will come an opportunity to confront him with some of his own stuttering.

(S) "*I-I-I-I* like this red car best."

(C) "Say I think I heard you bounce on a word there. Do you remember which one it was?"

(S) "No."

(C) "Well I thought I heard you go, *I-I-I-I* like the red car."

(S) "Yeah, I did. I do that a lot sometimes."

Perhaps this is as far as we would pursue this. If he has another moment of stuttering, then we can again ask him to tell us the word that gave him trouble. Of course, we wouldn't do this on every stuttered word. Far from it. We never nag. It makes no sense to teach the child to become highly aware of every little moment of stuttering but ask him after he has had some obvious stuttering. We are talking here about a repetition of at least three beats or a prolongation or an airflow blockage with some indication that he knows he is not moving forward. You will soon find that after only a few trials he will be able to tell you the word on which he stuttered.

As we continue we may wish to go deeper into this identification of stuttering.

(C) "*I-I-I-I.* Hey what did I do?"

(S) "You stuttered."

(C) "Do you remember what the word was?"

(S) "It was *I*, I think."

(C) "Yes that's right. But tell me more. What did it sound like?"

(S) "Well you kinda bounced on it like we talked about."

(C) "That's right I did. Could you do it like I did? Could you make it sound like mine did?"

(S) "I think it was kind of like *I-I-I* wasn't it?"

(C) "That's right, I went like this, *I-I-I-I.* That's very good. You are a good watcher and listener."

At this point the child is usually beaming from ear to ear. It is so much fun to be able to correct an adult.

This interchange might seem quite insignificant to most of us but yet much learning has taken place. The child has been able to see that someone else can stutter without becoming emotionally upset. He has seen somebody stutter and then casually talk about it. Stuttering has not been condemned as bad; rather it has been shown to be interesting. For a change the child has had a chance to correct someone else instead of always being the one corrected.

Great strides have now been made in our attempt to objectify stuttering. We have both confronted some stuttering with an objective attitude and without the shame, fear and embarrassment that usually accompanies it. The child has even been able to put some pseudo-stuttering into his own mouth. Until now stuttering has been a very unpleasant experience. But here in one short moment he has been able to produce stuttering at will and without any harmful side effects.

One other thing that clinicians might be concerned about is the child's continued use of the word stuttering. In these interchanges we made no attempt to correct him, because we have found that very soon now, he will probably start using more objective terms like, "bouncing" or "stuck" if these are the words we use. The more we talk about "bouncing" and being "stuck" the more he will tend to use those terms. As we have said before, stuttering is not an unmentionable word with us. We treat it like the word disfluency. Both are too general and vague for most children. Our aim should be to remove the mysteries and to speak in more objective and descriptive terms.

Making Stuttering More Voluntary

Now that he has done some pseudo-stuttering we can make a little game out of this activity.

(C) "Now let's see just how good a watcher and listener you are. I am going to do some talking and I am going to pretend to get stuck on some of my words. When you hear me getting stuck your job is to ring this buzzer and stop me. Then you must show me what it sounded like. For example to win a point you must ring the buzzer and say, 'you kind of bounced on it *li-li-like* this.' Now, if you don't catch me, then I get a point. Here's a red car and it has four *ti-ti-ti-tires* and it has . . . Hey, you didn't catch me that time. I said *ti-ti-ti-tires.* So I get a point. Here we go again. This elephant has a bi-bi-bi . . . (The child rings the buzzer.)

(S) "I caught you on *big.*"

(C) "That's right you did. But now you must tell me what it sounded like."

(S) "Well you kinda bounced like, *bi-bi-big trunk.*"

(C) "That's right so we will give you a point for catching me and for being able to show me what it sounded like."

When he is able to "catch" us and imitate our repetitions we then can move on to other types of stuttering. One of the reasons we do this is to give him a chance to stutter in many different ways. This helps him to learn that stuttering need not be completely involuntary. Most stutterers feel that something happens to them which causes them to stutter and they do not feel responsible for it. We must remove this feeling of helplessness. Also, imitating different forms of stuttering helps them overcome the fear of the actual sound of stuttering but the main benefit is that the child learns that he can exert some measure of control over his behavior, that he really is not helpless. For the first time he feels that he is controlling the stuttering rather than the other way around. Moreover, since he must consciously manipulate his mouth in order to imitate these different types of stuttering he will be better able to tolerate some of his own stuttering when we get to that stage of therapy.

Often in certain children we can immediately let him do some pseudo-stuttering in the game of "catch me", described above. Taking turns, we may then ring the buzzer and imitate him when he stutters. Surprisingly perhaps, many children enjoy this activity and certainly it will help them to reduce any fear, shame or embarrassment that may have begun to occur. What we are seeking is merely to make a beginning impact, to change some of his thoughts and feelings about stuttering.

Exploring the Emotional Nature of the Child

Let's pause here to point out that many other things are happening in the therapy session besides the above activities. We are still spending much of our time in play and conversation. We are also continuing to probe his concerns. Every child has other sources of stress besides stuttering and it is very difficult to treat a child's stuttering successfully if he is having serious trouble with other aspects of his life. So let us find out what these are. Although we are not psychiatrists often there is much we can do to alleviate some of the child's suffering. Often if we can just identify and talk about some of the other problems children have we will be helping him solve them. Perhaps we can help by having a parent or teacher make some adjustments after we discover something that is bothering him. We have witnessed surprising decreases in stuttering by such intervention.

Nevertheless our main concern is to learn more about the emotional aspect of the child's stuttering. What are his real feelings about stuttering? What are the reactions of others to his stuttering? Of course, we wouldn't just sit down with a child and begin firing questions at him. The probing can be very indirect but in every session, we try to find out something new about how he feels about his problem. We can blend our comments quite naturally into the flow of the play or conversation, phrasing them in such a relaxed and casual manner that the child is hardly aware that he is being questioned. Also, when doing this, we would be watching him very intently for any signs of discomfort. Is he trying to change the subject or ignore us? Is he showing signs of restlessness? Perhaps his body language tells us that the subject is still too painful to explore. Whenever we recognize any of these signals we usually back off and resume our playing. We never force him to discuss unpleasant material. Another day will come when the child has more confidence in us and can confide.

Here is an example of how we might proceed with a child in order to find out his family's reaction to his stuttering. (Again this might not take place during one session but be spread over a number of sessions.)

(C) "How about a few peanuts? I'm kind of hungry. (Some long silent pauses here while we eat peanuts.) A boy told me yesterday that sometimes when he got stuck on a word at home his mother would make him stop and try it again. What does your mom say when you have trouble on a word?"

(S) "Oh, she just tells me to talk slower."

. (C) "How about your dad, does he ever say anything?"

(S) "Sometimes he makes me keep saying the word over and over until *I-I-I* get it right."

(C) "Maybe he gets upset when you get stuck?"

(S) "I heard him say a bad word once when I got stuck. We were both in the garage and mom wasn't there. She would have been mad at him if she would have heard him. She doesn't like him to swear."

(C) "You know the trouble is, parents are older and they forget how hard it is for some kids to learn to talk. Sometimes they forget that we are trying our best to talk good."

In later sessions we might ask again about his parent's reactions to his stuttering and he may then have much more to say about it. Also we can explore the reactions of siblings, teachers, classmates and the children in the neighborhood to his stuttering. Often a child experiences great relief once these experiences are shared with a clinician who cares.

Again let us repeat that the information we get from children may not necessarily be correct. Many children will fantasize and give us completely false stories about what has happened to them at home, in school or on the playground. It would be folly to confront parents or teachers with things the child has said as if they were complete truths until we have checked carefully and perhaps not even then! Nevertheless, it is important that the clinician realizes that the wild untrue tales she hears, even if completely false, are reflections of the inner turmoil in the child, and so may be of extreme significance.

The following example illustrates why we need to be careful in condemning parents even in our own minds. A fellow clinician related this story:

It seems that one of her young stutterers told her about being, "slapped in the mouth by my dad everytime I stutter." The clinician was understandably shaken that such behavior still existed. She knew that something had to be done or else the child could get worse.

When she called the home and was telling the mother as diplomatically as possible the ill effects of such punishment on the child's stuttering the mother became outraged. "My husband never has nor never would do such a thing. How could you accuse him of such a terrible thing?"

After some fast talking on her part the clinician was finally able to calm the mother down enough to discover the cause of the child's fantasy. It seemed that the father had a habit of looking away everytime the child stuttered. The child had understandably taken this as a sign of rejection and had distorted the reality.

Yes, we must be careful in our judgments of condemnation. One of the ways we can be objective is to show interest in the positive side of the child's perceptions. How do people show their love and acceptance of him? What good things happened to him yesterday? And so on. His responses to this line of investigation may show that he has loving people who indeed care for him. Then we can help him understand his negative feelings and thus erase some of his distortions of reality. Unfortunately not all such children are fantasizing. Some parents are indeed guilty of wrong doing and cruelty. A few children are still being slapped and spanked because of their stuttering by well meaning but ignorant parents. A competent clinician can do much to help them understand that such behavior is unwise.

Exploring Struggle and Tension

Once the child learns to imitate your pseudo-stuttering we can proceed to teach him to locate and identify more precisely some of the things he does when he stutters. For instance he can come to recognize the different places in his mouth where he blocks the airflow. When a child begins to have these airflow blockages he usually will begin to show some real concern. They can be a devastating experience for a young child. He begins to have that helpless feeling of being stuck, that he is paralyzed and cannot move. For a moment time stands still. These blockages are frightening and we need to help the child understand what is going on. We must desensitize him to these traumas and help him learn to open his "speech doors" rather than shutting them tight.

We might introduce the subject like this:

(C) "Now I am going to pretend to get stuck on some words and it will be your job to tell me where in my mouth I got stuck. OK, here's the first one. The elephant has a long . . . (The clinician blocks the airflow on the *t* sound.) trunk. Now where did I get stuck on that word?"

(S) "You got stuck on the word *trunk.*"

(C) "That's right but can you tell me where in my mouth I got stuck? (The child shrugs his shoulders.) Did I squeeze my lips together too hard like on the word . . . (The clinician blocks on the *p* sound.) *paper?*"

(S) "No, it wasn't like that."

(C) "Did I get stuck down in my throat like on . . . (The clinician blocks on the *k* sound.) *candy*?"

(S) "No, not like that either."

(C) "Did my tongue get stuck up behind my teeth like on . . . (The clinician blocks on the *t* sound.) *table*?"

(S) "Yeah, that's how it sounded."

(C) "That's right my tongue did get stuck up behind my teeth on the word *table* just like on the word *trunk.* "

Often at this point you can have the child begin to do some experimental blocking in his mouth. If the child is still quite shy and defensive we would of course wait for a better time.

(C) "Here's another one. I have a yellow . . . (The clinician blocks on the *p* sound.) pencil."

(S) "It was on *pencil* and you jammed your lips together."

(C) "That's right. Now why don't you try it just like I did on that word *pencil*?"

(S) "(The child blocks on the 'p' sound.) Pencil."

(C) "Right. Did you feel your lips getting jammed together? It's like trying to drink from a bottle with the cap still on. Nothing comes out. So unscrew the cap and let the word come out. Do it again on *pencil* and this time feel your lips getting really jammed up then letting go." (The child does this and practices doing it on many other words beginning with different sounds.) "Say, that's hard work. Let's rest a minute. It's kind of scary when we get stuck and the word doesn't come out, even when we're just pretending. But we need to learn what it feels like so that we can make some of our words come out easier. It's no fun to be stuck and not be able to say a word."

We need to point out here that we haven't made any attempt to have him identify his own word or sound fears. Most children with mild stuttering are rarely aware of any sound or word fears and certainly no clinician wants to start him thinking about them. But aren't we making him more concerned about his stuttering by pointing out the different areas of the mouth where he may be blocking the airflow? The answer is no. Knowing where in the mouth he blocks doesn't cause anticipatory fears. It does however reduce the mystery and fear of stuttering when it occurs. We want the child to know what happens and what it feels like when he has these blocks and to recognize that he can do something about them.

Now that the child has learned to locate the site of the tension in his mouth we may move on to having him feel the differences between proper and improper tension:

(C) "Watch me say this word *pencil*. (The clinician blocks the airflow on the *p* sound.) What happened that time?"

(S) "You jammed your lips together."

(C) "That's right and then I squeezed them tighter. Can you show me how to put my lips together just right so that the word comes out easy? (The child says the word *pencil* fluently.) Good job. Let me try . . . *pencil*. There I brought my lips together loosely and the word came out easy. How about pretending to get stuck on the word paper? Don't say the whole word. Just get stuck on the first part. (The child blocks on the *p* sound.) OK, that's enough. Now put your lips together nice and loose but don't say the word until I tell you. (The child puts his lips together without excessive tension.) Are your lips together just right? (The child nods his head.) All right now say the word. (The child says the word *paper* fluently.) Now get jammed up on the word *bear*. (The child jams his lips together.) Put your hand up on your mouth and feel your lips squeezing tight. That's enough. Now put your hand up there again but this time put your lips together just right. OK, now say the word. (The child says the word fluently.) Fine! That's the way to do it. Now this time close your eyes and jam up your tongue on the word *table*. Don't say the word just jam up your tongue. Feel that? (The child nods his head.) Now keep your eyes closed but this time put your tongue up there loosely. Feel that? (The child nods his head.) OK, that's enough for today."

We would do this on many different sounds until the child becomes familiar with the proprioceptive feeling of both the proper and improper tensions.

These then are just a few of the procedures we would use if the child was having airflow blockages. Our aim has been to reduce his fear and remove some of the mystery which surrounds this traumatic kind of stuttering behavior. The child has learned the feel of both stuttering and fluency. We have not attempted to teach any modification but have only made him aware of the differences between stuttering and fluency. From past experience we have learned that a mild stutterer will choose the easier form of talking once he realizes he has a choice.

Reducing the Severity of Repetitions and Prolongations

Although the child has learned in our beginning sessions to identify and imitate some easy repetitions it is often necessary to go further. As with the techniques we earlier discussed concerning airflow blockages we need to make him more aware of both his severe stuttering behaviors and the milder, more fluent forms.

A case study in our district provides an example of how another clinician successfully treated a child simply by increasing the child's awareness of his numerous repetitions. This is what she told us:

Billy was five years old and had just entered kindergarten. The teacher, after a few weeks with Billy, was nearly frantic. She reported that his stuttering was so bad that it took him fifteen minutes to ask her permission to use the bathroom. After seeing Billy everyday for a week the clinician understood what the teacher meant.

Billy's stuttering consisted exclusively of mild repetitions which showed neither tension nor struggle. His attitude was also completely carefree. But what repetitions they were! When counting them the clinician found that there could often be anywhere from five to twelve repetitions per word and he stuttered on well over fifty percent of his words. So what was she to do? She didn't want to do anything that would cause him to change his carefree attitude nor the mild form of his repetitions but she knew sooner or later he would get penalized or frustrated by them.

At first the clinician was cautious and tried through play to develop Billy's trust but later she realized that this wasn't enough. His stuttering persisted and the other children were understandably beginning to react negatively to it. Their reactions would soon make his stuttering worse. So she gambled:

We will attempt to condense several days of therapy with Billy.

(C) "We have talked before about bouncing on words. Now let's count the times we bounce. First I will pretend to bounce and you count on your fingers how many times I bounced. The car is re-re-re-red. How many times did I bounce?"

(Billy) "You bounced on red."

(C) "That's right. But how many times did I do it?" (They played this counting game for awhile, taking turns doing the pseudo-stuttering.) "Now let's change the game. I am going to bounce four times. (The clinician holds up four fingers.) The tiger has a ta-ta-ta-tail. (The clinician counted on her fingers as she repeated.) See I did it four times. You try it four times. (The clinician holds up her fingers and points to each one as Billy has a pseudo repetition.) That's fine. Now you hold up as many fingers as you want and I will bounce that many times. (The child holds both hands up.) Ten. Oh, that's a lot! OK, here goes." (The clinician repeats ten times as Billy laughs with glee. They take turns at this game.)

As Billy began to succeed the clinician would occasionally ask for zero repetitions. Although Billy continued to ask her for large numbers of repetitions she was asking him for fewer and fewer and was amazed to find that he was even starting to speak fluently on demand.

The clinician would then occasionally stop Billy during their play and tell him that she had heard eight bounces on that word. Could he do it again with only two? This was done sparingly because she didn't want Billy to think that she was being overly critical and non-accepting of his stuttering.

The clinician was then taken ill and so was forced to stay home for several weeks. This upset her because she was afraid that all of their progress might be wiped out but she received a call one day that revived her spirits.

Billy's mother called and tearfully told her a miracle had happened. "He doesn't stutter anymore." The clinician tried to warn her that this was probably just temporary and that his stuttering might return but upon her return to work the clinician found that Billy was indeed talking fluently. In fact she couldn't get him to stutter. At first she was gentle with him fearing a relapse but later she put him in pressure situations and found that he just didn't stutter no matter what she did. Everyone at school was amazed. He has never stuttered since.

We do not agree with the mother that a miracle had taken place. There were several important factors that resulted in Billy's dramatic change.

The clinician had built a good foundation by establishing a warm and friendly relationship right from the beginning. Stuttering had been discussed openly, objectively and in a relaxed manner. Because Billy's problem was severe the clinician had to make him more aware of his stuttering than she might have done with a milder case but she did this in a nonthreatening way. Once Billy became more aware of his stuttering and was able to make voluntary variations of those long repetitions he realized that he could change the way he stuttered, that he could control it. This we feel was the crucial lesson he needed to learn.

His stuttering had been compulsive. He spoke a stuttering language. He felt that he had no choice but to speak repetitively and had resigned himself to talking this way. This was why he showed no signs of struggle. He never tried to change his speech patterns because he did not know he could change.

The clinician might have had trouble had she immediately tried forcing him to speak fluently. The child would probably have begun struggling and gotten worse. But her use of counting and varying the repetitions was done without threat. It was a fun game that the two of them played. As with many of these young stutterers we have known, once Billy realized he could choose and control the way he stuttered, that he was not helpless, he stopped stuttering. Extensive drill and long hours of therapy were not required. The impact of having a choice was the critical factor. He no longer felt helpless.

We would recommend the same kind of therapy with a child whose stuttering consisted of long prolongations. Again we would do some pseudo-stuttering in which the sound or its silent posture was held for varying lengths of time. Let us illustrate:

(C) "Watch me a minute. I am going to hold a sound until my fingers touch. (The clinician raises one finger from each hand and holds them about five inches apart.) I have a s------*ister*. (As the clinician stutters on *sister* she moves her fingers together at a slow speed. When they finally touch she says the word.) What happened to my fingers when I said the word *sister*?"

(S) "They started to move."

(C) "That's right. And what happened when they touched?"

(S) "Then you said the word."

(C) "Right. Now let's play a game. You hold your two fingers up just like I did and, when I start holding onto a sound, you slowly move your fingers together. I must hold that sound until your fingers touch. When they touch I will say the word. Let's try it. The elephant has a *l*--------*ong* trunk. (The child moves his fingers slowly together.) Now it's my turn. I will hold them this far apart and you pretend to get stuck on the word *watch*. Remember you can't say it until you see my fingers touch."

(S) "W------*atch*."

(C) "Hey, you didn't hold it long enough. You didn't wait until my fingers touched. Try it again. (The child succeeds this time.) Now it's your turn. Hold your fingers as far apart as you want and I will hold the word *shoe*. (The child holds his fingers as far apart as possible.) That long! All right. Don't forget to move your fingers. *Sh*--------------*oe*. Wow! That was a long one!"

These then are some of the activities we would use with a child who is prolonging. We attempt to lower his anxiety and fear through the use of the fingers and pseudo-stuttering. Then we attempt to vary the length of the prolongations. Once we teach the child to vary his stuttering we can gradually reduce its length. When the child discovers he can change his stuttering patterns the stuttering will usually begin to recede. We have reversed the morbid growth of the disorder and when this occurs, fluency returns.

Conclusion

Quite often with these mild stutterers this is as far as we will need to go. These few simple activities, the fluency builders we talked about in the preceding chapter, the parent and teacher contact, the warm and relaxed attitude on the part of the clinician and the desensitizing work on his emotional experiences are often all that is necessary to reverse the course of the child's stuttering and make him fluent.

Again let us emphasize that the speech activities are not as important as the attitudes that we have helped to change. If we remove some of the mystery, help him to understand some of the basic features of his stuttering, build up his fluency, he will heal himself. Because stuttering is not yet a fully developed problem requiring great effort to eradicate such an approach is remarkably effective. Over and over again we have been amazed at the ease with which this change occurs in a young child. Our job is simply to find the key which makes his stuttering understandable and nonthreatening. Of course, each child is different and one never really knows in advance exactly what key each stuttering child needs to discover. It seems that at some point he understands what is happening and stops struggling. We have had children go home and tell their mothers, "You know why I stutter sometimes? It's because I bounce on my words." Or they may say, "I squeeze up my lips too hard and don't let the word come out. That's why I stutter." Once this insight has occurred the stuttering begins to disappear. The understanding of what he is doing and the realization that he doesn't have to do it, as he has always done it, seems to be enough. Recovery rarely comes overnight but there seems to be little doubt that progress is being made.

The more experiences we have with these mild stutterers the more we have come to realize the importance of our intervention. We greatly aid them in their understanding and in their ability to do something about their stuttering. Perhaps they might have attained normal fluency on their own without our help but certainly we made it easier. We also know that without our help many of them may not make the transition to normal speech but instead will become severely handicapped and serve as a life long reproach to our competence.

The Confirmed Stutterer

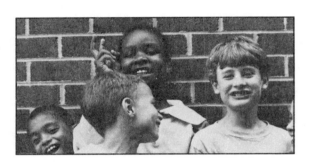

The Confirmed Stutterer

Now let us move further along the continuum to consider the child whose stuttering is a definite handicap. Obviously he shows a large quantity of stuttering some of which can at times become quite severe. This is the child that you dread seeing if you have any doubts about your ability to work with stutterers. Because he certainly needs help and people will be expecting you to treat him.

Most clinicians seem to equate the confirmed stutterer with the coming of maturity, that somehow no one becomes a true stutterer until he reaches adolescence. In our experience this is just not true. We have worked with many children as young as four years old whom we would classify as confirmed stutterers. Since it is not our intention to get into any theoretical or semantic arguments, let us explain what we consider a confirmed stutterer.

Such a child has speech that is characterized by repetitions that often last for more than five beats. These repetitions sometimes rise in pitch or loudness. They are frequent and come at different places in the sentence, not just on the first word. The confirmed stutterer of any age tends to show signs of struggle and tension when he speaks. There may be facial contortions or other secondary characteristics resulting from his struggling. Often he will show some hurt or fear or shame although this is not always the case for some of our young confirmed stutterers seem to show little concern about their stuttering. He often blocks the airflow on many of his utterances and these blockages may become so intense that he gets red in the face, blinks his eyes or jerks his body around.

Another child may have very little overt stuttering because he has already learned how to hide it by postponing or avoiding words on which he feels he may have trouble. Or he may simply back up and start over like this: "I want the *rrr* . . . *ah ah* . . . I want *ah ahm* . . . well I *ah* want the car the red car." We hate to see this behavior occurring because it will be hard to help him face his stuttering. We will need to spend a lot of time helping him touch his stuttering before beginning to modify it.

But let us not spend any more time on the characteristics of the confirmed stutterer. It has been our experience that most speech clinicians know when they are faced with such a stutterer. The problem is not in the diagnosis but in the treatment.

We begin therapy with the young confirmed stutterer much as we did with the mild stutterer. Beginning slowly and indirectly we gradually move to a more direct confrontation of the stuttering. Once again the speed with which you proceed should depend entirely on the child's readiness. If you are proceeding too fast his behavior will soon tip you off. With some reservations we feel that proceeding slowly is usually wiser. Remember that this child needs time to get acquainted since both of you will be exploring his stuttering together. He will need time to develop trust if he is to reveal his stuttering or his feelings about it to you. Nevertheless don't proceed so slowly that both of you get bored or lose track of the fact that there is a job to be done, not merely to play and have fun. We must always be ready to move swiftly when a child gives us the opportunity but also be willing to slow down or wait when the child's reaction so indicates.

As we did with the mild stutterer we usually begin by commenting on some of our own little pseudo-stutterings, then his. Later we discuss some of his moments of real stuttering objectively, exploring together some of its general characteristics. With the mild stutterer this is often all we needed to do but with the confirmed stutterer we must go further.

The Three Ways of Saying Words

After some general exploration of stuttering we usually start talking about the three ways that one can say a word, the fluent way, the hard stuttering way and the easy stuttered way. Here is an example which will demonstrate the use of these three ways:

(C) "Now John, let me talk for awhile. We are going to learn about the three different ways of saying our words. One way is the regular way. If I was to say a word in the regular way it would sound like this, 'watch' (The clinician points to her watch.). Now there is another way I can say that word, 'wa . . . (The clinician blocks the airflow and struggles a little.) *wawawatch*'. Whew, that was hard. That is called the hard way of saying a word. This is the third way, '*wwwwatch*' (The clinician makes an easy effortless prolongation or repetition.) and that was the easy way."

"Right now you try to say all your words in the regular way but sometimes you get stuck. Saying words in that easy way isn't so bad. Whenever we get stuck on a word instead of saying it in the hard way we are going to learn to do it in that new easy way. Kids that learn to stutter in that easy way don't get stuck so much and later they tell me that more and more of their words start coming out in the regular way. All that's hard to understand right now, but we will practice it."

"Now let's play a little game. I will say some words and it will be your job to tell me if I said the word in the regular way, the hard way, or the easy way. 'Watch'. Was that the regular way, the easy way or the hard way? I'll do it again. 'Watch'."

(S) "Regular."

(C) "That's right. How about this one? *'Ta . . .* (blocks airflow) *TABLE'*. Which way was that?"

(S) "The hard way?"

(C) "That's right. I really got stuck hard on that one, didn't I?" (We usually do more examples of these two ways so that he can get them straight before trying a word in the easy way.)

(C) "How about this one? *'YYYellow'*."

(S) "Hard way."

(C) "Oh, I tricked you on that one. Listen again, was it in the hard way? *'YYYYellow'*."

(S) "Well, you sure stuttered on it."

(C) "It wasn't the regular way was it? But was it the hard way like this, *'Y* . . . (The clinician has a hard block on 'yellow'.) *'YaYaYellow'*?"

(S) "No, it wasn't that bad but you still stuttered on it."

(C) "That's right, but remember about that easy way we talked about. Listen again. *'YYYellow'*."

(S) "Yeah, that was more easy."

(C) "That's right, I didn't get all squeezed up did I? I just kind of *Illet* it out easy just like I did there on *'Illet'*. Did you hear that one?"

(S) "Yeah, you didn't hold your breath or anything."

We use this little activity for a few minutes every session until he is able to identify all three ways correctly.

(Let us mention a couple of things here before we go on. It is important that the clinician is the one doing the stuttering in this activity, not the child. First it shows the child that you are not ashamed of stuttering and so sets the tone of learning to be objective about stuttering. Children in the beginning are sometimes quite unwilling to confront their own stuttering. It is much easier for them to look at and evaluate the clinician's stuttering. If you do some first he will be more willing to show his stuttering after seeing you. We have a private rule in our therapy: we never make a child do anything that we haven't done first.

An interesting note about the above therapy excerpt was the child's determination to call any little disfluency stuttering. After the clinician's pseudo-prolongation on the word "yellow" the child said, "Well, you sure stuttered on it." That particular moment of stuttering was no more severe than what any normal speaker has on occasion, but to this child it was stuttering. Perhaps this is partly why he didn't outgrow his disfluency. Or, possibly, since becoming a confirmed stutterer he has acquired an almost fanatical interest in perfect speech. What a shame he didn't get some therapy when he was younger. Early therapy is so important. Who knows, perhaps we could have straightened up some of his misconceptions at an early age and he wouldn't have progressed to this more advanced stage of stuttering.)

The next step in using the three ways of talking is to get the child to do the three kinds of utterances deliberately, to say a word fluently, to stutter hard, and to stutter easily on it. This teaches him to evaluate his speech behaviors. And of course, it helps him become desensitized to his stuttering. Now let's return to another example a couple sessions later.

(C) "Well, I can't trick you any more, I guess. You can always tell me which one of the three ways I am using. So now we are going to do something different. It is your turn to say some words and it will be my job to guess if you said them in the easy way, the hard way, or the regular way. Ready? How about this one?" (The clinician holds up an elephant.)

(S) "That's an elephant."

(C) "That was the regular way."

(S) "Right."

(C) "How about this one?"

(S) "That's a kangaroo."

(C) "Regular."

(S) "That's a car."

(C) "Regular. Hey you are doing all regulars. How about some other kinds? Like can you do this word "table" in the hard way?"

(S) "*Ta* . . . (He puffs out his cheeks, blocks the airflow and gets red in the face.) *TABLE*. (He finally blasts the word out.)"

(C) "Whew. You sure got stuck!" (They both laugh.)

(S) "Yeah, I really got that one stuck."

(C) "Was that a real one?"

(S) "No, I just pretended like you told me to." (The clinician realizes that the original task was too difficult so she changes her plan and tries to get him to imitate her use of the three ways.)

(C) "All right now, let's do it a different way. I will say a word in one of those three ways and it will be your job to say the word just like I did. If I do it in the hard way, you make one in the hard way, just like me. I see the *ca* . . . (blocks the airflow) *ca-ca-car*. Let's hear you do that."

(S) "I see the *ca* . . . *ca-ca-car*."

(C) "Did I say it in the hard way?"

(S) "Yes."

(C) "Did you say the word in the hard way?"

(S) "Yes."

(C) "That's right. *ThThThThe* (very easy, short prolongation) alligator is green."

(S) "The alligator is green."

(C) "Listen again. I made a word in the easy way and you didn't that time. *ThThThThe* alligator is green. What was my easy word?"

(S) "The."

(C) "All right see if you can say the word 'the' like I did?"

(S) "I don't know how."

(C) "Like this. (The clinician holds two fingers about four inches apart and as she makes the prolongation she moves them together slowly.) What happened when my fingers touched?"

(S) "You said the word."

(C) "That's right. Now you try it. Watch my fingers." (They both prolong 'the' as her fingers move together. When the fingers touch they both say the word.) "Now let's see if you can do one by yourself. Watch my fingers."

The clinician now goes through a series of words using the three different ways. On the easy words she sometimes uses a little prolongation; on others a short repetition. Now that he is learning to imitate her properly she can begin again to let him do them on his own.

(C) "Now how about making the word 'watch' in the easy way?"

(S) "*WWWWatch*."

(C) "Good, that was nice and loose. Now you give me a word and tell me whether to say it in the hard or easy way."

They go back and forth giving each other words and telling how they should say them. As you can see she had to change her plan with him. He wasn't able to start doing these easy words right away as some of our clients do. She had to proceed more slowly with him. The clinician had first to show him how to make those easy words by using her fingers to demonstrate a prolongation. (Any other physical way that you can use to demonstrate what you want his mouth to do helps a great deal.) Then she was able to give him some commands to say words in one of the three ways. Often she had to help him on some of these until he began to get the idea. It was only then that she was able to go back to her original plan and have him say words using the three ways.

Now that you have taught him to identify and produce the three ways of saying words you will be able to use this knowledge in the future. Whenever you talk to him about a stuttered word you have some common ground for understanding each other. Since all stutterers have the cure to their malady already in their own mouths you can point out some of the easy stuttered words that he has in his speech that up till now he has not recognized. It is a rare stutterer who doesn't have some easy stuttering in his speech, but these are usually ignored and the stutterer doesn't realize that they occur. All that he notices is the hard stutterings. An example might sound something like this:

(C) "Hey, stop for a minute. Did you know that you just had one of those easy words? You said, 'I *lllike* the red car'. You made that word 'like' in that easy way that we talked about. Did you know that?"

(S) "No."

(C) "You see, you are already starting to make some of those hard words come out easy and you didn't even know it. Anyway, I might interrupt you again when I hear some more of those."

We draw his attention to these easy words for several reasons. First, this will help him to be more aware of the positive things he is already doing and it might encourage him to do more easy stuttering words. Secondly, you thereby give him some hope. Perhaps things are getting better and this speech teacher can help me! Thirdly, we are making progress in the area of desensitization.

Locating Tension

In addition to practicing the three ways of uttering words, we also work on identifying his actual stuttering behaviors. We want him to know what is happening when he is stuttering. We did this same procedure with the mild stutterers and we do it also with the confirmed.

Once again we don't over-analyze but we do want him to know where in his mouth he got stuck. The clinician can best teach this new knowledge by doing some pseudo-stuttering on a number of different words. Both she and the child will then attempt to discover the location of the tension. Perhaps the tension will be bi-labial as in "paper" or lingua-alveolar as in "table". Remember to demonstrate words beginning with different sounds so that many areas of tension will be explored. Usually the child will have trouble locating the point of tension unless he also makes a pseudo-stuttering on the word. Encourage him to do this if he isn't able to locate the tension of your stuttered word. Later you will have him do the pseudo-stuttering and then tell you where in his mouth he stuttered.

(C) "How about pretending to stutter on the word 'table'?"
(S) *"Ta . . . TaTaTable."*
(C) "Where in your mouth did you feel something get jammed up?"
(S) "My tongue got stuck on the 't' sound."
(C) "Yes, that's right. Where was your tongue when it got stuck?"
(S) "I don't remember."
(C) "All right try it again and see if you can feel where your tongue gets stuck." (The child stutters again on "table".)
(S) "My tongue got stuck up behind my teeth."

Once the child is able to identify the tension during pseudo-stuttering then we can begin to ask him to go through the same process on a real stuttered word. Often after a particularly hard moment of stuttering we may interrupt him and have him go back and explore what happened that caused him to stutter. When we begin interrupting a child like this we are careful not to do so if he is talking about something important or emotional. At other times when we do interrupt him we need to empathize with him about being interrupted.

(C) "For the next few minutes I will occasionally interrupt you after you get stuck on a word. Being interrupted is no fun but if we are going to make talking easier we must learn what is happening to you when you stutter."

This is a most important phase in our therapy. The child is learning to reach out and touch his stuttering. This enables him to see that stuttering is a physical event that can be felt and experienced without fear or pain. The negative emotions that foster stuttering grow in

69

the darkness of ignorance and irrationality and they cannot tolerate the light of observation and confrontation. When the child can confront and examine his stuttering he begins to break the grip that stuttering has on him.

Cancellation

Now that he has learned about hard and easy stuttering we can help learn a new and better way of stuttering on words that he has just stuttered on. All of his life people have told him to say a stuttered word over again but they always made him do it fluently. For the confirmed stutterer this is too big a jump. Besides he knows how to say the word fluently. What he doesn't know is how to stutter without abnormality.

Our way is to teach him a better way of stuttering, an easier way, one that won't trouble him or others. Fluency will come when he learns he need not be helpless, when he finds he doesn't have to struggle or avoid. The reader should recognize that as with all our stutterers we are trying here to return the stuttering to an earlier, milder form. We want to turn the calendar back to the time when his stuttering consisted of mild repetitions and prolongations. Here is an example of how we might proceed:

(C) "Now I am going to get stuck on some words in that hard way. You pretend to be the speech teacher and stop me whenever you hear me getting stuck in that hard way and then show me how to make it come out easier. Now be careful not to stop me when I make one come out in the easy way. Only stop me when I get stuck in that hard way. OK. You're the teacher now."

"Well teacher, yesterday after school I . . . (The clinician blocks the airflow.) I went . . . Hey, why didn't you stop me? Didn't you hear me get stuck on that word 'I'?"

(S) "Well, yes, but I forgot."

(C) "Now remember you stop me and show me how to do it in that easy way so that I can learn a better way." "I went home and changed into *mm . . . mmmy* old . . .

(S) "Hey, you got stuck hard on that word 'my'."

(C) "Well, teacher, I didn't mean to. How can I say it better?"

(S) "Say 'my'. 'My old clothes'."

(C) "Yeah, but sometimes when I try to say it perfect like that I get stuck hard."

(S) "Oh yeah, say *'mmmmy'* like this kind of slow and smooth like that."

(C) "Well, let me try that . . . 'my'." (The clinician says the word fluently.)

(S) "No, make it easy like this 'mmmy'. See you just kind of stutter on it like that but it's not bad stuttering, see?"

(C) "OK. *MMMMM* . . . (The clinician has another hard block.)"

(S) "No make it more easily. Don't squeeze it so hard. Like 'mmmmy', see?"

Then we will take turns being teacher, children like this and it really helps them learn. Often we have found that children can learn a concept better when they try to teach it to us.

So we have another good activity to help us return the stuttering behaviors back to an earlier, milder form. Also, it helps them understand what they must aim for in the future. We are not after fluency right now. That will come later. Instead we are interested in creating an easier form of stuttering. But you can also see in this example the pressures most children have to be perfectly fluent. When he corrected the clinician the first time, he showed her how to say the word fluently instead of the desired easier way. It takes a lot of work to get these young stutterers to see that first we will make our stuttering easier and then the fluency will come. Children are no different than adults in this respect. They want fluency now, even though it is obvious that the step from stuttering to fluency is too great.

Changing Stuttering to a Milder Form

Now we are ready to move forward again. This involves taking a moment of hard stuttering and turning it into the easier form.* What we are attempting to do is to modify a moment of stuttering right while it is happening. This isn't easy but it can be taught and learned. It means that the child must confront his stuttering behavior head on and then make a conscious effort to manipulate his mouth in the direction of easier utterance. This is why we stressed earlier the learning of the three ways of uttering words. That is why all of the work we have just outlined is so important. We need to provide a good foundation so that this new task might be learned with less difficulty.

We might introduce this step as follows:

(C) "Let me show you something. See this pencil? Watch what

---

*With adults we often refer to this as pull-outs.

happens to it. (The clinician closes her hand around the pencil and tries unsuccessfully to push it up through her clenched fist.) Why can't I push the pencil out?"

(S) "Because you have your fist too tight."

(C) "That's right. I am squeezing my fist so hard that I cannot push the pencil through. That is very much like a word that you get stuck on. The word is like the pencil and your mouth is like the fist. Sometimes when you squeeze up your mouth too hard the word just cannot come out. Now watch what happens to my fist when I try to say a word. This is my wa . . . (The clinician tries to push the pencil through her clenched fist as she is having some hard stuttering. As she gradually begins to loosen both her mouth and fist the pencil and word come out slow. *'WaWaWatch'.* Can you tell me what happened?"

(S) "Well, when you loosened your fist the pencil could come through."

(C) "And what about the word 'watch' that I was stuck on?"

(S) "Well, it started to come out when you loosened your fist too."

(C) "That's right, it was like my mouth was doing what my fist was doing. Watch again. When I squeeze up my fist I am going to squeeze up my mouth, and then when I start to slowly loosen up my fist, I will loosen my mouth at the same time. See the *'wa* . . . (The clinician blocks the airflow and clenches her fist.) *wawawatch'.* (As her fist loosened so did her mouth and the word started to come out slow and easy. She continues to do this for several words until he is getting the idea.) "Now this time I am going to squeeze up my mouth and start doing some hard stuttering. When I do, you make a fist. Then when you loosen your fist I will loosen my mouth and let the word come out nice and easy. Are you ready? Let's try it."

"Here's an elephant and it has a long *tr* . . . (blocks the airflow). Hey, you are forgetting to clench your fist. Let's try it again. Here's a *ka* . . . KANGAROO. (The word explodes out because he has sprung open his fist too quickly.) You see, you opened your fist too fast and the word really popped out. Now remember to make your fist loosen up slowly so that I can make my mouth loosen up slowly too. Let's try it again."

"The hippo is *bi* . . . *bibig.* Say, that was more like it. Did you hear how nice the word came out? I got stuck real hard but I changed it into a nice, slow and easy one. Let's do it some more."

They go through some more words until the child begins to understand. Often once they realize that we must stutter for as long as they want they sometimes hold their fist closed for an eternity. But we grin and go along with them. It is great fun to torture the speech teacher in this way. A child has little opportunity to get back at all the adults in his world. But when they do hold us in a block for a long time we should come out of it laughing and out of breath. They should see that the experience of stuttering for so long did not frighten us. We could laugh about it. Laughter and fear cannot abide one another. So besides teaching him new ways of stuttering we are also helping to relieve some of his emotional distress.

Easy Stuttering for Clinicians

This process of loosening the mouth and letting the word out slow and easy is relatively simple on a word like 'watch' which begins with a continuent sound. The clinician gradually loosens up her mouth and then begins letting the 'wa' sound come out gradually and smoothly. Some refer to this as a prolongation or 'sliding' the word out. But what about a word beginning with a plosive sound like 'table'. This is a bit more complicated and will require you to do some practice at home. Through using the word 'table' as an example we will demonstrate how it should feel when you change it from a hard to an easy stuttered word.

When you are stuttering hard on it you will feel your tongue jammed up against the alveolar ridge. You will also feel air pressure building up behind your tongue. The air wants to escape but you are forcing it back with your tongue. Now gradually loosen the pressure on your tongue by reducing the force of the air pressure pushing up against it. Then gradually begin to relax the tension you have purposely placed on your tongue. When you remove some of this lingual pressure you will probably hear a little burst of air escaping between the tongue and the alveolar ridge. You then need to change these bursts into a small steady stream of air. Once you have this steady stream of air it is easy to add the voicing necessary and once again 'slide' into the word. But beware of prolonging the vowel. It should be *'tttable'* not *'taaable'*.

Putting the process down on paper makes easy stuttering appear quite complicated but if you will try it, you will find that it is really quite simple. In fact your young stutterer will usually start doing it automatically when he tries to make the word come out slow and easy. Returning to our therapy session, the clinician continued to demonstrate this technique on several words until she felt that the child was getting the idea. In this way, we can teach him how to release himself from his hard blockings. Of course, this is only practice for learning a new skill, but this practice is needed if we are ever going to help him learn to change real stuttering into a milder form.

Some problems occur, as they always do, no matter what is done. Just recently a clinician was telling us about the success she was having with a young stutterer. He had gotten the idea of making his stuttering easier by slowly loosening his fist at the same time he was relaxing the tension in his mouth and for the first time he was learning to change a moment of stuttering. In fact his classroom teacher told the clinician of the sudden improvement not only in the severity of his stuttering, but also in his willingness to take a more active part in class activities. "But," said the teacher, "everytime he stutters on a word he doubles up his fist."

The clinician was upset. Had she made his stuttering worse by creating another secondary characteristic? Although the stutterer probably would have gradually discontinued the use of his fist once he became more proficient in reducing the tension during his stuttering, the clinician was determined to extinguish this behavior immediately. So the next day when he came in she had him watch her fist while he had some pseudo-stuttering on a word. Then on the next word she had him change the hard stuttering into easy stuttering without watching her fist. To her surprise he did this with ease. In fact by the end of the week they never talked about or used the fist again. From then on the idea of changing from hard to easy stuttering was understood and the physical example was no longer needed.

Now that we have learned all of these skills when using pseudo-stuttering during practice sessions we can begin doing some modification of speech in real situations.

Inserting Easy Stuttering into Real Speech

One of the things that we do is to have him learn to insert some of these easy, mild stutterings into his regular speech. This helps the client in many ways. First, he learns to voluntarily manipulate his mouth during speech, thus heightening his awareness of what his mouth is doing. Second, the act of doing something voluntary while speaking tends to reduce his fears of talking. Finally, the new easy stuttering is providing him with a good model of the goal behavior that we are seeking.

There are many ways that you can devise to teach him how to

insert the easy stuttering purposefully. You may underline some words on a reading passage. These underlined words should be uttered in that easy stuttering way. (We try to underline only those words we think he will say fluently.) Or you may touch him on the arm to signal that he is to stutter easy on a upcoming word, keeping your hand on his arm until he has easy stuttering on a word. Then remove your hand and wait until he says a couple of sentences before using it again. Sometimes we give him a hand signal and keep signalling until he has an easy stuttering. Of course, we let him teach us first. When he gives us the signal we do the easy stuttering. Then later we take turns giving signals to one another. During this activity we are not concerned with any of his hard stuttering that might occur. The only time we would mention it would be if he had a particularly rough time on a word. Then we might stop him and talk about the word. But our main interest at this time is getting him to change words voluntarily during normal communication.

The Use of Physical Contact

We need to make some comment here on the use of touching with our clients. Clinicians must be careful not to infringe on the rights of the client. Some children react unfavorably at first to a clinician's physical contact and we should be alert to this. Although many clinicians feel that they have the right and should touch every child whenever they wish, it is our belief that children have the right of privacy. We have observed clinicians who (after feeling a client become tense after some physical contact) have asked the child where they might touch them. Some children have asked to be touched on a sleeve or other item of clothing. The clinician should respect the child's wishes in this matter.

This goes far in gaining the child's respect for us. Later as we take turns touching each other during speech activities we find that the children lose their apprehension about being touched. This gradual change is healthy and part of the client's increasing trust in us.

We saw this demonstrated so well while watching an older white clinician working with a young black child. She was having some problems because the boy held some deep seated resentments concerning race. She had observed some of her white colleagues touching and hugging this boy although she had the feeling that he was despising them for it but being forced to accept it.

During the next few weeks she was careful to respect his privacy but she still kept trying to find ways to initiate more physical contact that might be acceptable.

When playing with some toys she made sure that their hands would touch occasionally. She made it seem casual and accidental. She pretended not to know how to jump rope and had him show her. She didn't get it right until he placed her hands on the rope and jumped with her.

These, along with many other similar actions helped the child to lower his defenses enough to enable them to have a good clinical relationship. It was a lot of work, but his stuttering was reduced as the relationship developed. Later, when evaluating her eventual success, the clinician felt that they would have failed if she had rushed or simply ignored the physical contact.

Now let us return again to our discussion of easy stuttering. After he is able to insert an easy stuttering word on our signal we have him count the number of easy stutterings he has without getting a signal from us. We might decide on a certain quota before we can quit and go on to something else or we might try for a certain number in order to win a peanut. The activity might be introduced like this:

(C) "For the last few days we have been learning to make some of our words in that easy way. Now today we are going to change that a little. I am not going to give you a signal today, but I am going to keep track of how many of those easy words you can do on this little counter here. So now your job is to tell me how to play baseball and we will see just how many of those easy stutterings you can make." (He starts to talk and has an easy stuttering on every word.) "Hey, wait a minute. Slow down. Your doing it on every word! (They both laugh.) You outsmarted me that time. They were all good easy words, too, by the way. But that sounds funny when you do it on every word, doesn't it? It sounds like a robot talking. Now let's start over and this time just do one every once in awhile. One every sentence would be just fine."

A few children might not use any easy stutterings at all. If this happens then we simply point out to them, once again, what they are supposed to do. If this doesn't work, then we can go back and do some more signalling until he gets the idea.

There are any number of activities that you can develop from this idea of helping him insert easy stuttering into his speech. You can both have counters. He counts your easy stutterings and you count his. Sometimes you must remind him that he is doing too many but this isn't much of a problem usually. The important thing is that he is teaching his mouth a better way of stuttering.

When we first started using some of these techniques we were amazed to find that without our even mentioning it the children were beginning to make some of their hard stuttering easier. We had planned to teach them how to make a moment of hard stuttering easier at some later date, but they were doing it without our even talking about it. It seems to come naturally. As children begin to learn this easy way of stuttering they unconsciously begin changing their hard stuttering to the easier form.

Many of our clients who started modifying the stuttering on their own were not aware of it. After questioning them we became convinced that this was a totally unconscious phenomenon. They were not aware of doing anything different on their hard stuttered words. These were the children who had many easy stutterings in their speech even before therapy. It was as if the body has the cure just waiting for the child to discover it. So when we give him a little extra training and sensitivity the body is able to help cure itself as it does with so many other disorders.

Changing Hard Stuttering During Real Speech

Unfortunately not all children get free speech so easily so we must move on. The next logical step is to teach our client how to change that moment of hard stuttering during live ongoing speech.

This is a difficult assignment for any stutterer and we must realize what we are asking of him. We are requesting him to confront his fear and stuttering behaviors directly and to be able to make some conscious manipulation of his mouth right at the moment when his difficulty is greatest. This is why we have postponed this activity. Hopefully, we have developed some trust and the child has learned not to fear his stuttering quite so much. But the clinician should be prepared to have him fail many times during this assignment. It is not vitally important how many times he can successfully make his stuttering easy. What we seek is the self knowledge that he CAN make his stuttering easy, the realization that this is possible. The day that he discovers he can voluntarily do something about his stuttering will change his life. That is the day when stuttering loses its powerful hold on him, when he need feel helpless no longer. He has faced his fears and won.

This is how you might begin to teach him how to make his hard stuttering easier during real speech:

(C) "The last couple of days we have pretended to get stuck in that hard way then before we finished saying the word we have changed it to the easy way. Now we will try to do that same thing but this time we're not going to pretend. Sometimes when I hear you getting stuck on a word, I am going to touch your arm like this. Whenever you feel my hand on your arm, your job is to keep jammed up on that word on purpose. Then when I take my hand away you can start making the word come out slow and easy. So when I touch you, you just keep stuttering hard on the word. When I let go then make it come out easy. Here, watch me. I am going to start talking now and get stuck hard on purpose. When you hear me get stuck you touch my arm. I will stay stuck until you let go." (The clinician lets him touch her a few times until she thinks he understands.) "OK. Now it's your turn. How about telling me about some of the things you see in this picture." (Make the conversation something as concrete and as free from emotion as possible. It is better not to have him extemporize at first. This is a harder form of talking and his assignment is tough enough as it is.)

(S) "Well, there's a man washing windows and one mowing the *llll* . . .(The clinician reaches over and touches him.) *llalalawn.*"

(C) "Stop a minute. You forgot to hold onto that word until I let go of you. This is really a hard assignment and many times you will forget and make mistakes. You have to be brave because it takes a lot of courage to do what you are doing. That old stuttering is pretty scary stuff and it takes a tough guy to fight it. So let's try again."

(S) "There's some *ki-ki.*" (The clinician touches him again and he holds the word but it blurts out as soon as she takes her finger away.)

(C) "Say, that was better that time. You were able to hold onto that word until I took my finger away. You're a pretty tough kid. But now remember that you are to make it come out slow and easy. That time you popped it out like this. (The clinician demonstrates.) So let's try again."

(S) "The kids are swimming in the *po* . . ." (The clinician touches him.)

(C) "Now hold that word. Keep stuttering hard on it. Now start to make it come out nice and slow. (He is able to make 'pool' come out easy.) Hey, you did it. You fought that word until you made it give up." (They are both happy and laugh together. She puts the picture card away and they sit back. Perhaps she gets out the peanut jar.) "That's enough of that. Let's have some peanuts."

"You know, I had a kid last year about as old as you at another school. And he stuttered bad, worse than you do. He started to get a whole lot better after he learned to make those hard stuttering words come out in that easy way just like you did a minute ago. He said it was like riding a bucking bronco. You've got to stay on it until you can calm the horse down and make him go where you want him to. Just like with one of those hard words. You have to stay with it and fight it until you can make it come out nice and slow and easy."

Here at last we have come face to face with the stutterer's greatest fear. In the beginning of therapy we talked about and demonstrated stuttering. Later we confronted the sound and feel of the disorder through the use of pseudo-stuttering. Now we have reached the center or core of the stutterer's fear. The mouth is unwilling to move or if it moves, it does so uncontrollably and spasmodically. Because of this fear stutterers develop the secondary characteristics that we associate with the severe stutterer. And the difficult aspect of this confrontation is that we are asking them to not only face the fear head on, but also to remain in that dreaded confrontation until the fear can be reduced enough to enable the stutterer to modify the word. In the past he has either avoided the word altogether or stuttered on it as quickly as possible. Once he has stuttered then in effect he has escaped his fear and gotten relief. So we are asking him to change so much more than just the mere stuttered word. We are asking him to change all of his learned responses to his greatest fear. But when he does accomplish this task there is an automatic reduction in struggle and other secondary characteristics which results in a natural increase in fluency.

We always quit on an activity like this as soon as we get a success. The impact was made and doing more would only diminish the feeling that he has at the moment. Tomorrow there will be time to further develop his skill and insight.

Carryover is another reason we don't drill excessively. The techniques become something associated with the speech teacher and the speech room. We try to keep speech class as much like the outside world as possible. We try to make the class a part of the flow of the child's life.

Now that he is learning to modify some of his real stuttering we can begin to have him do it voluntarily and without prompting.

(C) "During the last few days you have been learning to change some of those hard words into easier ones. But today I am not going to touch you when you have a hard word. Let's see if you can do it on your own. Now here's your assignment. For the next five minutes try to talk as good as you can but when you have some hard stuttering on a word, then try to make it easier. Now I will hold this counter and keep track of every time you do. Do you think you could remember to do it at least one time in five minutes?"

(S) "Oh, I could do it at least ten times."

(C) "Now wait a minute. That's a lot of times. Let's see if you could get at least three. All right, begin."

We like to have him help us in setting the goals. His prediction was probably unrealistic at first, but we made a compromise which will probably be about right. In any case he will learn that it is harder than he thought and will become more realistic in the future. Having him help set his own goals involves him in the teaching process.

We do many variations of the above activity. You can have him take the counter and check himself. This enables you to see whether he is aware when he does the task successfully. Or we may have a contest to see who can change more hard stuttered words. There are many ways of helping him learn that he doesn't have to surrender when stuttering hits him.

It should be understood that as we do these speech activities we continue our investigation of the child's emotional and psychological needs. Though we have already discussed these needs in the previous chapters we would like to point out that the confirmed stutterer probably will have experienced more emotional suffering because of his stuttering and so we must spend more time and effort in this area. (Once again, this may not always be true. Some young confirmed stutterers seem to be little affected by their stuttering. Their struggle and avoidance seem almost automatic and without much accompanying emotion. Usually, however, this changes as they get older because stuttering doesn't go unpunished or unstigmatized for long. All stutterers will suffer eventually if they live in our society.)

Getting Parents Involved

It is at this point in therapy that we often use a parent to help us. Before using a parent you must feel quite sure that he or she will be a reliable helper. Parents, because of their great love, can sometimes become overzealous in their helping activities and can cause great harm to the child and spoil all your efforts.

This reminds us of a tragic story told us by a school clinician. She had a boy with a mild language and articulation disorder. The parents were intelligent and seemed anxious to help in any way they could. So the clinician suggested some little activities that they could do over the summer. The clinician told them that a few minutes a day would be sufficient.

In September she was horrified to find the boy stuttering severely and the parents angry and upset. They had spent as much as two hours a day helping the child talk better only to find that he was beginning to stutter. Then, when he began to stutter, they worked even harder but it just made him worse.

This clinician said she would never again make suggestions of this nature right before summer vacation.

Even after you feel confident about a parent's judgment you should still quiz the child on the results of his parents help.

Nevertheless, some parents can be valuable helpers, mainly by being able to remind the child to use the easy speech that we have been practicing. In order to do this we have the parent come in and teach them about easy stuttering. In this conference, both you and the child should teach the parent how to stutter easy. We do this so that the parents can actually see and feel the difference between the hard and easy forms of stuttering. And be sure to explain the need to reverse the growth of the disorder. Tell them that first the child must learn the easy way of stuttering and only then can we begin expecting an increase in his fluency.

We have seen many children have fun in these parent sessions. At first the parents look and feel a bit foolish as they practice stuttering in different ways. For once the child has a feeling of superiority over the parent. He seems to feel that, "It's not so easy to stutter is it?" It is good for the parents too. They begin to realize that stuttering isn't as simple as they thought.

After we give the parent an experience on how to stutter we can then talk about what they can do in the home to help their child's stuttering. Sometimes we work out a signal which will indicate to the child that he is having a lot of hard stuttering that he is disregarding. He can then try to change some of them to the easier kind. With other parents we just ask them to use the word "easy" whenever the child is having a particularly hard time with his speech.

That is about all that we want them to do except to give the child extra loving and support. We do not ask them to give other commands or advice. The word "easy", spoken softly and without threat is often enough.

We must also make sure that the parents understand that this help is only to be provided occasionally. We don't want the parents to encourage the easy stuttering all the time. The child will quickly come to resent both the parents and the clinician if this happens. A reminder now and then from a parent can be a big help in the therapy process.

Building Fluency

In the chapter on the borderline stutterer we mentioned the need to do some fluency building every day. We also need to do a lot of this with the confirmed stutterer. We must create opportunities and conditions so he can be given a chance to be fluent everyday. Indeed, while we are attempting to reduce the severity of the stuttering we should also be building up the fluency he does show and making it stronger. This becomes more important as the disorder becomes milder. When it is apparent that the severity is being reduced through therapy we can work harder on building up the fluency.

You can also begin to put the child under more stress now that he is talking easier but we never put more stress on him than he can handle successfully. If we start increasing the communicative stress and he begins to have some bad stuttering, then we stop and talk about it and see if we can't solve some of his difficulty. If after returning to the stressful communication he is still not able to handle it, we drop the task for the moment and return to this activity at a later date. This rarely happens in our experience. After a number of these retrials he should be desensitized enough to handle the stressful situation.

Many of our little stuttering clients seem to be better able to handle communicative stress after therapy than their normal speaking peers. Children have told us that their friends didn't know how to call up a store and ask for information. This is a new experience for most young children. Very few second graders have ever called up a store to ask how much their skateboards cost. Such an experience makes your client feel more mature and you are exposing him to speaking situations that he will have in the future.

By this time your client should be showing marked reductions in both the quantity and severity of his stuttering. He should also be able to talk openly and candidly about his stuttering. So we try to find out about any trouble spots he might have. Is there any person to whom he still has a hard time talking? Are there any situations that have provoked much stuttering during the past week? Are there any words or sounds with which he has had some particular problem? When we find these special problems we will try to invent ways of being able to work on them in therapy.

Building Independence

Finally there comes a time when you begin to consider dropping the child from active therapy. He is talking very well and needs a chance to go out on his own for awhile. The progressive course of the disorder has been reversed and although not completely fluent, both the quantity and the quality of the stuttering have been greatly reduced. Although he may still have an occasional hard stuttering he has a new self confidence in his ability to control the movements of his mouth. Also he is usually so happy at this point about his speech that further therapy is usually nonproductive. His talking is much improved and he wants a chance to enjoy his new freedom. It is time to give him some time off.

Another reason we recommend releasing him for awhile is so that he can have the chance to take the final step to fluency on his own. The advantage of this speech vacation is that some of our stutterers have reached higher levels of fluency on their own and thus have the feeling that they have "cured" themselves. When they say so, we are happy. We have come to have no fear of regression with these children who feel that way. A child who thinks that he has "cured" himself is so full of confidence that we doubt whether stuttering would ever have a chance to start up again. But if it does reappear, usually you can plan to work with the child again at a later date. When you release them for the first time you can consider this just the end of the first phase of therapy. You may go through many phases before you can release the child for good.

Complete change seldom comes from one learning experience. As in most living things, change in stutterers is not a continual or straightforward process. Rather it moves forward cyclically. Spurts of progress are followed by temporary lapses into disfluency but always the general trend is toward fluency. Do not keep these children too long. If you do, they will begin to depend on you for their newfound fluency.

When we first started in this job as a public school specialist in stuttering we made the mistake of keeping some children too long in therapy. We wanted to make absolutely sure that they were "cured". As a result they became fluent only when we were still seeing them and whenever we dropped them they would have a relapse or when summer vacation came they would start stuttering again. Finally we realized that we cannot protect them forever. We must send them out with some flaws so that they can gain the strength they need.

Some children need no further therapy at all. A few need booster sessions. Usually after dismissal we manage to see the child again after about a month. Usually he will be very glad to see us whether he is having trouble or not. A few are rather depressed, concerned because some of their old stuttering has returned. The stuttering is not as bad as before but he has again become afraid. Once you reassure him that this is normal and all part of getting better, he calms down and you can talk about his problems. Often he has forgotten some of the things we have taught him. He will tell stories about stuttering real badly on some word. We must get him to start being objective again and to analyze what happened. In some pressure situation he has probably panicked and started to force out his stuttering in his old, hard way. But it is amazing how fast his skills come back.

After a week's booster session the child is usually talking well again. Moreover he has grown considerably from the experience. He has gone out on his own and has learned something new. He has experienced some success and some failure. He now knows much better the kinds of things that will put pressure on his new found fluency. During our week of booster therapy he has learned how to be a better problem solver. He will also have more confidence because he has seen his stuttering return again but has been able to do something about it.

Although we have no rule of thumb we often schedule another therapy session in a couple of weeks to see if the progress he made during the week long booster session has held. Then we will not see him for another month. So it goes until we are seeing him perhaps once a year. We keep giving him more and more time between visits. He will continue to grow in strength and confidence. We must remember once again that it is not our job to cure him. We just try to change the course of the stuttering, to return it to a milder form. The child ultimately does the rest. And they do!

Working with Parents

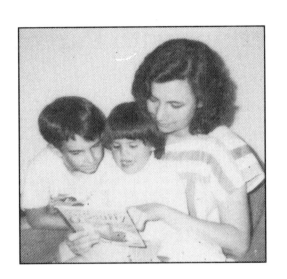

Working with Parents

One of the problems working with stutterers in the schools is that we cannot devote as much time to the parents as we would prefer. Often we are lucky to see the parents even once or twice in person and then keep them appraised of developments via the telephone. This has been our usual method of dealing with parents although with some of the severe stutterers we have managed to arrange further appointments during the course of therapy. Or if a child tells us of some inappropriate or dangerous parental behaviors we will try to make more than one appointment. Many might take this to mean that we are advocating minimum parental involvement. This is just not true. The reason is simply a matter of time and necessity. Also in many homes both parents work adding to the difficulty of scheduling conferences. Most public school clinicians will understand why this regrettable situation exists. However, we should all avail ourselves of every opportunity to see parents more often. Their influence on the child is so much greater than ours that maximum parental involvement should always be a foremost concern.

We have had some very good experiences with parents during the intensive summer programs that we have offered to a small number of our clients. Since school was not in session the parents had to bring the children to us. This created an excellent opportunity to work with the parents as well as the child. These programs ran for six weeks, five days a week and we would see each child for thirty minutes. During many of the sessions we invited the parents to come in and take part in therapy. The first few times we would just have them watch us working with their child. They were able to see how we interacted with the child, that we were nonjudgmental and relaxed in our therapy. They could see that we treated stuttering openly, honestly and objectively. We also wanted them to see how we played with the child, allowing him to direct much of the activity while keeping our questions to a minimum. Hopefully the slow, easy pace of the session would give the parents a good example to follow.

After the parents became more comfortable with us we gave them a more active role in the sessions. We might ask them to play together with us and found that they often adopted our way of playing and our slow rate of speech. With a few we had them help us locate the areas of tension on some stuttered words. Or we would all do some pseudo-stuttering on a word and then locate the point of tension. Sometimes we might produce pseudo-repetitions varying the number of beats.

We found that our stutterers generally progressed much faster during these summer programs and we must assume that one of the reasons for this was the increased involvement of the parents. So if you have a chance to see parents more often, we would strongly recommend that you do it. But if you cannot see the parents as often as you would like, perhaps some of our experiences here can help accomplish more during your limited time.

One of our goals in the parent conference is to acquire information. We wish to know all we can about the child and about his stuttering. There are two ways that you can get this information. One way is by direct questioning and the other is a more open, indirect approach. In our experience the indirect way is far superior.

If possible we try to ask a general question in the hope that the parent will use this as an opportunity to unburden themselves of some of their pent-up feelings of frustration, guilt or anxiety resulting from their child's stuttering. Asking the parents these large general questions makes for a much better interview. As parents begin talking they often will tell you things that they hadn't intended to reveal and say things that they had never brought to their own consciousness before. Besides there are often significant bits of information that parents want to tell us but which will not come out if the situation becomes a question-answer session. Asking questions such as: When did Johnny start to crawl, walk, talk, or stutter. Only elicit short answers. The parents never get a chance to unburden themselves and as a result we fail to gain any insights about our client. The parents need to talk and talk freely and we must conduct the interview in such a way as to make this possible.

You might use lead-in phrases such as: "Tell me about Johnny. By that, I mean what what kind of a child is he? What are some of his strengths and weaknesses, his likes and dislikes, etc.?"

Another general question one might use is simply to ask them to tell you about his stuttering. You might begin by saying, "Now how about telling me about his speech development. Go right back to when he first started to say words."

As they are telling you the story of his speech development you can ask specific questions during their narrative, such as, "When did you first start to notice his stuttering?" "What do you think might have caused it?" You can also ask at this time what they have done to help him get over his stuttering. "I'll bet you've had lots of advice from relatives and friends? It seems that everyone is an expert on the problem of stuttering and they all feel that you are not using the right methods to cure his stuttering. People love to give advice to us about our children." Be sure to pause here because sometimes parents have a lot of pent-up hostilities concerning advice from others. Or we might ask: "In what situation does he seem to stutter most severely? Often supper time or right after school seem to be the worst times." Of course, even with this indirect type of interview we will still be asking and answering questions as we go along but it is more like a conversation than a cross-examination. It is both friendly and informative. We make sure that the parents understand that we are not condemning or making judgments, that we are simply trying to understand the problem.

Our interviewing techniques are much like those we use in therapy. We are trying to get the parents to talk and to talk openly. So we often use the reflective type of speech, reflecting back the parent's words. This shows that we have gotten the message, are interested and it encourages them to talk further. Also we are continually forcing ourself to tolerate pauses. Too often we tend to fear and avoid these pauses. Perhaps we are afraid it will show others that we have nothing to say or that we lack knowledge. But the pause is an effective way of getting the parent to talk further. After all, they don't like to be interrupted or lectured to anymore than we do. During a pause the parent might be deciding whether to tell us something meaningful. They often need time to build up their courage and they need to feel that we will give them a chance and not make judgments on their revelations.

For this type of interview to be effective we must show our respect for the parents. If they are to talk openly with us they must feel at ease. We try to make it clear that we are exploring, not trying to assess blame. "Please help me to understand so I can better serve your child."

We are also interested in knowing about the child's relationships with his siblings and his neighborhood peers. How have they reacted to his stuttering? Does he have other deviant behavior such as nail biting, bed wetting, etc.? Finding out about the child's daily routine is also important. We have found many instances of a child's time being overly structured. Sometimes the stuttering seems to be a call for help to let him be free to grow in his own way.

We will not soon forget a little boy who showed many other nervous behaviors besides some mild stuttering. Upon asking the parents about his daily routine we found that his day which began at 6:30 a.m., was almost continually structured until his bedtime at 7 p.m. In addition to his school he had church catechism several afternoons a week. He had Bible studies and verses to memorize. There were youth meetings and other activities at the church. He had music lessons and the resultant practice during the week. He took swimming lessons and was on a little league team. We were convinced that he had loving parents, parents who were trying to provide every possible activity which would benefit him. But when they began to tell us of his daily activities they began to look more and more upset as they continued. Finally, the father stopped and began talking about actors and other famous people who had nervous breakdowns due to over-work. "I wonder," he said, "if we are hurting our son with all these activities?" Then the mother spoke and said that all of the activities were important and she couldn't see how any of them could be discontinued. Then they asked our opinion.

One is always tempted to shout out something about giving a child ulcers by the age of ten, but this would accomplish little and only antagonize them. So instead we said something like this:

"I don't claim to be a child psychiatrist, but I do know something about how to help children who begin stuttering. Talking is hard work for some children. Most of us don't realize that unless we have tried to learn a foreign language. And your boy is showing us that he is having trouble making some of his words come out fluently. It is also a time in his life when he is learning many other new skills. So I would suggest that you try to make life as simple and uncomplicated as possible for him. Relax the discipline and give him as much freedom as possible. You discovered this just now as you were talking about your son's many activities. When describing them you began to feel uneasy. You started to realize that slowly over a period of time his weekly activities have been increasing until now he has little or no free time left. But please don't feel that this means that you are bad parents. Just the opposite is probably true. You love him so much that you want to provide him with all the possible opportunities for learning. But during this time when he is trying to learn so much it will probably help if you drop some of these planned activities and give him every possible chance to outgrow his stuttering. The more we uncomplicate his life the better his chances are of outgrowing it. When he does outgrow his stuttering, then you can gradually

return to the kind of discipline and after-school activities that you think are appropriate. We would therefore recommend that you try something different for a few months to see if it will help him with his talking. It has been our experience that this kind of change in a boy's life will often bring back the normal fluent speech."

After this we tried to steer the conversation around the joys of being a child, the fun of being free and without responsibility. We felt that the point was made without hurting their feelings. They felt that they were the ones who discovered their error and did not feel condemned or made to feel foolish.

Just a postscript to this episode. We found out later that they had told their pediatrician about what we had recommended and that he had agreed with us. And only then did they decide to take our advice. It is a bit ego deflating at times to realize the difference in credibility between us and members of the medical profession, but the important thing is that the parents did institute drastic changes and with them the child just blossomed. His school teacher marveled at the remarkable change and the boy overcame his mild stuttering problem in a short time.

Besides seeking information which helps us to learn about the child, we should always try to alleviate the guilty feelings the parents might have. Although many parents appear calm and cool when talking about their child's stuttering, most have deep feelings of guilt. Society still generally feels that the parents are to blame for the child's stuttering. And parents feel acutely not only society's accusations, but also their own self condemnation. Every parent makes mistakes.

Some will disagree with our desire to remove parental guilt because in many cases the parents are indeed guilty of doing fluency-harmful things to their child. Our response is that the events which might have been harmful to the child have already happened. They are ancient history. We must be concerned with the present and future if we are to help the stuttering child. If they are listening to their guilty feelings they can't listen to our suggestions. Also, parents will always be more willing to tell us the full story of their dealings with the child if they feel less guilty. And finally, a guilty parent cannot do us or the child any good in terms of the future.

The parent's guilt can also affect the child. Often he may feel that he is the cause of their distress and so in turn he may feel ashamed for letting his parents down. There are so many evil ramifications concerning guilt that we must deal effectively with it.

How can we help to reduce parental guilt feelings? One important way that has already been mentioned is through the type of atmosphere we create during the interview, an atmosphere of objectivity and exploration. This is a big help to parents. Many of them come to us worried sick about what we might say to them. When they see that we are friendly, objective and noncondemning much of their guilt will already start to recede.

Another way is to empathize with the parents about some of their unspoken feelings. When talking about stuttering you might ask them to tell you what they do when the child stutters. Most will reply that they ignore it or give the child some little piece of advice. Don't comment right away on the appropriateness of their response. Try instead to verbalize some of their negative feelings. You might say something like this:

"It must be really hard for you to hear him talk that way. You feel so helpless. We all want our children to have an easy time growing up and talking seems so simple to us. Why must he struggle so? Some parents have told us that they feel so frustrated because they don't seem to be able to stop the stuttering no matter what they do. The stuttering gets so bad that sometimes you just want to plug your ears!"

Many parents interrupt us at this point (If they don't, we have a long pause in order to give them time to respond.) and either burst into tears or start talking rapidly giving vent to their frustration. Others breathe a sigh of relief. At last someone understands. No one has spoken to them before about how much it hurts them to hear that "ugly" stuttering. People have blamed them but no one has spoken of their suffering. Many have talked to us about the unfair way in which they have been judged by those around them. Still others have confessed to hating their child's stuttering so much that they want to scream at him to shut up.

To all responses we must give as much understanding as possible. Parents must realize that they are having normal human feelings, natural feelings which they shouldn't feel any shame about. What we try to do is to see if we can't help them to accept and understand their feelings and to teach them as much as we can about what they can do to ease the child's problem. But just our accepting will help both parent and child tremendously because if the parent is feeling these negative emotions, the child is too.

Speech clinicians should realize that most parents come to the interview to get information rather than to give it. Encourage their questions for their questions will often tell us more about the stutterer and his family than our cross-examination.

The first thing that we can do is remove some of the mystery surrounding the stuttering. If we can demonstrate different varieties of stuttering to parents they can begin to understand what is happening to their child. Few parents can describe their child's stuttering. Some of them will give a general description such as: he repeats words or he gets caught on words but they are usually completely unable to describe their child's stuttering in any detail. We must demonstrate different kinds of stuttering and ask them to tell us if the child has ever had similar ones.

In demonstrating different kinds of stuttering we explain what is happening. Then we may imitate some of the child's stuttering and explain what happens then. Rarely we have even had the parent try to do some stuttering following our instructions. When they do this, much of the fear and ignorance that has always surrounded stuttering will be reduced. This will go a long way in being able to help them to listen unemotionally to their own child's stuttering. But many parents can't or won't do this pseudo-stuttering. We never force them and are always alert to any signs that may indicate that they're not yet ready to try any pseudo-stuttering on their own.

Discussing the Cause of Stuttering

Since one of the first questions we will be asked is about the cause of stuttering we try to be first to ask this question. We need to know what they think. Their answers are important for they tell us much about the kind of parents we are dealing with. We have heard parents use many different reasons for their child's stuttering. "He started stuttering right after his uncle Ernie tossed him up in the air and he came down on his head." "It started after he had the flu real bad." "It started because he didn't want to go to school." Or the parents may point to a death in the family or of a pet. They may blame the stuttering on the birth of a sibling or some other event which altered the family unit. They may tell us that he caught "it" from the older boy down the street.

The responses that parents give usually fall into one of three categories. They may blame an external event, or they tend to blame themselves, or they may not be able to answer the question at all. Those in the last group may respond like this:

"We have thought about this a lot. We have gone back and tried

to remember if we did something to trigger it or if some event happened to start his stuttering, but we just cannot come up with anything. We have tried to be good parents and love our child very much. We have tried to bring him up like the other kids. We just can't understand what went wrong."

If the parents blame an external event we accept their opinion without passing judgment on it. Sometimes it will be difficult to keep a straight face as when a parent told us that: "Johnny caught the disease from the little neighbor girl." But we try gallantly to show respect for their opinions. And we do have that respect since no one is sure about the exact cause of stuttering, we cannot with assurance rule out any possibility. Secondly, the particular cause of stuttering which they expound may serve several purposes: (1) It may relieve them of some deep feelings of guilt they harbor. (2) Since stuttering is so mysterious, a cause, no matter how bizarre, may satisfy the need to reduce that mystery. Some people are frightened by any uncertainties. We do not want to antagonize nor humiliate them so we listen acceptingly. Therefore, we might respond to parents who blamed the stuttering upon an external event like this:

"That's interesting and it might indeed be one of the contributing causes. Usually there are many reasons that cause a child to stutter. We don't know your child that well yet, but if he is like some of the other children we see then probably some of these reasons might help explain why he started to stutter or that make the stuttering worse." (We then go on to explain some of the causes of stuttering in other children.)

To parents who tend to blame themselves we attempt immediately to relieve them of some of the burden they bear. You might say:

"You know in the past the common practice was to put all the blame on the parents but we are now discovering that there are many other possible reasons. We see children who stutter from every walk of life, from loving homes as well as broken homes. We have children from rich and poor, large and small families. There seems to be no one reason that a child starts to stutter."

"Surely you have had a big influence on his life. And I'm sure that you have made mistakes. We all have. But you could bring up another child in the same way and he wouldn't stutter! Why does one child start to stutter while others don't? (We will then go into some of the causes of stuttering that will tend to take away some

*of the blame and guilt that they feel, The important thing is to
give immediate absolution for any sins of commission or omission
that may have occurred.)*

Many of the parents who say they don't know the cause of their
child's stuttering are really secretly blaming themselves. Parents
justifiably or not take most of the blame or credit for their child's
behavior. So we assume these parents feel some measure of blame for
their child's stuttering and we attempt then to give them a chance to
share these feelings with us.

Parents will usually want to know our opinion concerning the
cause of stuttering. This puts us in a rather tenuous position. The
problem is that no one seems to know for sure the exact cause of
stuttering. But the parents are waiting for us to answer and our
answers are important to their judgments of our competence. If we
try to avoid the issue or speak in generalities they will think we are
unknowledgeable. So even though the leaders of our field have no
specific answer to the question we must come up with something
that will satisfy the parents."

After hearing the parents talk about their views on the cause of
stuttering we might say something like this:

*"I wish we could tell you the exact cause of stuttering. If we
knew, then perhaps we could be done with the problem forever.
Unfortunately we haven't been able to find any one cause of
stuttering. But we have learned something about stuttering during
the hundreds of years that speech scientists have been studying the
disorder."*

*"One fact that is important to know is that talking is a very
complicated set of motor skills. Imagine what a hard task talking
must be for a child just learning! Scientists tell us that speaking is
the most difficult act of fine motor coordination that man must
learn. Let's take the sentence, 'I went to the store'. My jaw,
tongue and lips are all moving at a rapid rate and every movement
must be timed perfectly. All of this rapid coordination must also
be timed with the air coming out of the lungs."*

*"Another complicated skill the child must learn is knowing the
right words to use, putting them in the proper order and pro-
nouncing the words correctly. What really amazes us is that more
children don't have trouble learning to talk. Many parents have
told us that they have never looked at talking this way. Talking
seems so easy and comes so naturally for them. They get an idea
in their mind and open their mouth and out comes the right words*

effortlessly. But for a child just learning, the process is much more complicated."

"Now let's look at the reasons why some children seem to talk more easily and more trouble-free than others. If we took five children out to the playground who had never tried to jump rope before and gave them each a jump rope and told them to watch us so they could learn how, one or two of them would probably pick up the technique right away. A few more would struggle but after a time they would begin to have success. But there would probably be one child or two who just couldn't seem to master the coordination. This doesn't mean that the other kids were smarter or faster learners. What it means is that we all have different talents and abilities. What is easy for one is hard for another and vice versa. So it is with talking. Some children seem to learn the coordination of speaking faster and easier than others."

"Now, let's go back again to our one little child who couldn't seem to jump rope. If the child really wanted to learn he would probably take the rope home and try practicing alone in the back-yard. He might still have trouble but he would start getting the idea at least some of the time. If he kept practicing he would gradually improve until at the end of a week he would probably be jumping as well as the other kids. But what would have happened if we had hovered over him and tried to correct him after each attempt? He would probably start trying too hard and tensing up his muscles. And the harder he tried the worse he would do until in a little while he would probably give up in disgust."

"This is much like talking. All parents want to help their child learn to speak as fluently as possible. His mistakes bother them and so they do things that make him try harder. They do this not because they are mean or bad parents, but because they love him and want the best for him. But not only the parents, but the grandmothers, relatives and even next door neighbors want to help the child learn to talk as perfectly and quickly as possible. Just like with the jump rope, the child often will become tense and frustrated and therefore have a harder time learning."

"But this tension and frustration which is so damaging to easy learning can also be brought on by the child. All of us occasionally have some trouble talking and so he may say, 'I-I-I-I-I wwwwant a glass of water'. Although he had never thought too much about stuttering before, this particular morning he thinks to himself, 'Why didn't I say that right? Why can't I talk as good as Mommy

and Daddy or some of the other kids? Something is wrong!' And so he begins trying too hard. If that child who couldn't learn to jump rope right away had responded in the same way and began to put pressure on himself to be as good as the other kids he would probably never learn to jump rope. What happens is that the more he worries about not doing well the harder he tries and the worse he does."

"But in any case the major thing that we are concerned about is not the cause but what can we do to help him. We are not that concerned with what caused the stuttering originally. That is ancient history. What we need to do is to find ways of helping him to feel less pressure so that he can begin to break that vicious circle he is in. Let's discover the things that make talking difficult at certain times."

What we have tried to do is give the parents a simplistic analogy to the complicated question of the cause of stuttering. The real value of our reply was that the parents now have a more logical, understandable and unemotional explanation of the cause of stuttering. People often need concrete reasons for circumstances, in order to deal with the future. And, as we told the parents, we strongly believe that the original cause is unimportant at this stage of the child's development, since he is already stuttering. Nothing we can do will ever be able to return the child back to the time when stuttering first began. Our concern must lie with the present stresses and ways of alleviating them.

Just one last comment about our response to the parental questions concerning the cause of stuttering. We have never given the above answer to anyone. This reply was simply illustrative. With some parents there may be a need to get much more technical; with others we would answer the question with a few simple sentences. As with everything in this business respond to each according to their needs and abilities.

What the Parents Can Do

If our contacts with parents are to be productive, we must realize that they come to us not only to provide or get information, but to find out what they can do at home to help the child. It is essential that they carry away with them at least one or two fairly concrete suggestions or they will feel let down. They want very much to contribute something to their child's improvement but they don't know how. And there is no better way to alleviate guilt that to get the parents involved in the healing process.

One way the parents may be able to help is to occasionally use some restimulation. When the child has had a hard time getting his message out reflect back fluently the content of his utterance. This is the same process as the reflecting or echo type speech that we talked about with the borderline stutterer. This will tend to reduce the memory of stuttering and will help the parents listen to the words rather than the way in which they are spoken. Along with these better listening skills they can try to look at the child when he speaks even when he stutters. This shows their interest in what he is saying instead of signalling him that they are alarmed about his stuttering.

We also may recommend a short play period during the day where the child is allowed to direct the activity. We attempt to arrange an opportunity for the parents to watch us as we work with the child so we can show them how to conduct this play period. The chances for real learning are so much greater when the parents have an opportunity to see our words put into practice. We have an opportunity to demonstrate permissive, child-directed play and to show the relaxed way that we respond to his stuttering. The parents can see how we talk slower and simpler (although remembering to keep it natural) in order to provide better models. We are good listeners and allow the child to do most of the talking. And we are nonjudgmental. If the child has cars that fly we go along with his fantasies. We shouldn't correct the child and tell him that cars can't fly. This need not be a long period of time. The important thing is to do a little each day of this quiet and unhurried play.

With older children this play period can be a quiet, unhurried time over milk and cookies. A time for the parents to listen rather than always asking. If the child doesn't feel like saying anything that is his right. Other days he will feel the need to talk. And if the parents create that kind of atmosphere during this short period then the child will learn that he has this time. He will want to talk because he will not be hurried, criticized nor corrected.

Most of our children have a particularly hard time when they are excited. Many parents complain about this and wonder what they can do to help the child during these times.

First of all we usually give an example of a normal speaking child who tries to talk while under some emotional stress. Sometimes we use this illustration when talking to certain parents:

> *"Let me tell you of an experience that happened just the other*

day. My little girl, Sara, who has never had any trouble talking, fell off her bike and ran in to tell me about her accident. She was all excited, out of breath, and was sobbing a little when she said something like this, 'Da-Da-Da-Daddy I-I-I-I fell dow-dow-dow-down.' Then she gasped for air."

"Here was a little girl who never had a bit of trouble before this, yet she was talking, 'stuttering' all over the place. Now just think how difficult talking must be for your child when he is excited or under emotional stress!"

"When I saw that she was having trouble talking I told her we would go into the kitchen and get a glass of milk and then she could tell me all about what happened. Once we got in the kitchen and she got her milk she had a chance to catch her breath and relax a little. Then when she talked she only had one or two words that she got mixed up on. I did not interrupt her nor ask her questions about the incident. This was hard because I wanted to know all the details but I let her tell her tale in her own way and in her own time."

"At other times I have made the mistake of letting her tell me right away what happened and sometimes I have even interrupted her by asking for further details because I was excited too. But this seems to make talking harder for her for she gets even more upset and confused. Let's try not to demand speech of a child when he's emotional."

"I think your child would benefit from this new policy. During the times that talking is difficult for everyone we must be particularly careful with a child who stutters. I have learned to think in this way; if Sara can walk into the house under her own power then she probably won't require immediate medical attention. So I have time to sit down and listen quietly."

"Now, of course, you will not do this every time your child stutters. This is just for those few times during the week when he is so excited that he just can't seem to get anything out."

This little story serves well to get across the point. If we can give parents something to help them cope with these bad situations we will have helped both them and the child. This type of response also helps them to get the idea of removing stress from speaking. Many will find also that following a few of these suggestions will gradually make a change in their overall handling of the child generally as well as when talking.

Many clinicians have trained parents to be observers for them in the home. The parents are told to keep a diary on the child and then report their findings back to the clinician. They are told to hunt for pressures or situations that seem to increase stuttering. When they have noted a few of these they are instructed to call the clinician so that they can work out plans for reducing these fluency disruptive behaviors.

In this diary they can also note the situations that seem to be stuttering free. The parents are then encouraged to allow the child as much time in these activities as possible.

When parents begin being better observers they will notice that the child's speech will go in cycles. On the days when he is more fluent they should attempt to encourage more talking, while on his non-fluent days they should decrease the opportunities for talking without the child's awareness. One parent for example remembered that the child never talked much when they played together with the erector set. The child always seemed so intent on his work that he didn't have time to talk. This became a good activity for his non-fluent days. By playing with the child the parent demonstrated her love for the boy and the activity also was a good way to reduce the child's amount of speech. Other parents have gone on bike rides since this activity often reduces the amount of speech.

Parents also need to know that stuttering is a progressive disorder which may get worse with time. Mainly we alert the parents to recognize signs of struggle and tension. These may be blockages of airflow, facial tremors or body movements. We also have them watch especially for avoidances of certain words or situations. When the child begins using avoidances he has learned to be afraid and embarrassed because of his stuttering. The evidences of fear are a warning to us that the stuttering will probably get worse. In this connection the Speech Foundation of America (a group dedicated to the treatment and prevention of stuttering) has a little book which is often useful. It is entitled *If Your Child Stutters.** It tells parents some of the danger signals that they should be aware of. If they notice any of these danger signs or see anything new in the child's stuttering they should call us.

Some parents have made important changes in the communicative environment of the stuttering child because of these observations.

*For your copy, write: Stuttering Foundation of America, P.O. Box 11749, Memphis, Tennessee 38111.

As they begin to see the kinds of situations and forces that bring on stuttering in their child they make the necessary changes so essential to fluency. At the same time through their close observation they have also seen the actions and situations that promote fluency and so they try to increase the use of these activities. Parents of this caliber are thus able to change their lifestyle enough to bring about an end to their child's stuttering.

Certainly more could have been written about the clinician's interactions with parents. We have not chosen to do so because the literature on the subject of parent counselling is quite extensive and this one chapter could have evolved into the subject of another book. Hopefully the reader has gotten a feeling for the way we interact with parents. The specifics of the interview are quite secondary to the overall philosophy of respect and understanding that we have tried to create.

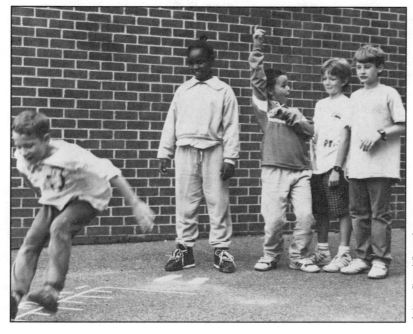

photo credit: paul diamond

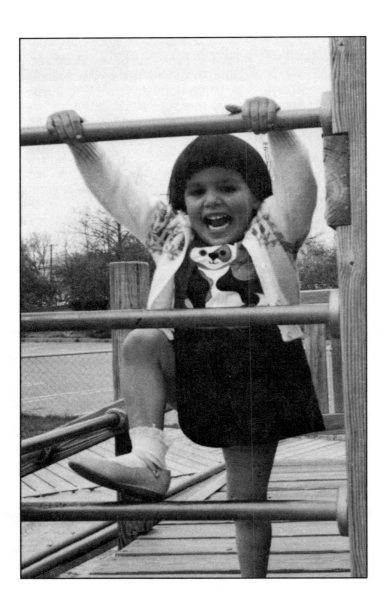

Working with Teachers

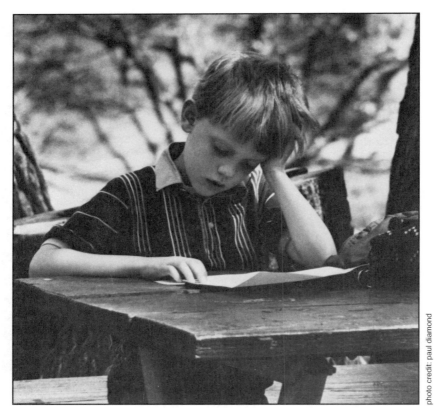

Working with Teachers

Teachers should play an important role in the remediation process. Since they have a big influence on our client we need to make every possible effort to work closely with them. Unfortunately, as with parents, we cannot see teachers as often as we would like. But we try to see them as much as possible. The friendlier we are with teachers, the more we get to know them, the more willing they will be to follow some of our suggestions.

Although not always possible we have tried to set up a half hour initial meeting with the teacher. We have found this more productive than trying to see them during recess in the teachers lounge. The teachers lounge has too many distractions for good communication so we try to schedule a meeting where we can have some privacy. After this initial meeting we find that we can communicate with teachers during recess because earlier we have had this quiet time together.

Much of our counseling techniques with teachers are quite similar to those we use with parents. We begin this short, private session by having them talk about the stuttering child. We tell the teacher that we are interested in knowing more about him. We ask her to describe him to us. Our aim is to ask general questions in order to get the teacher talking. The teacher needs to realize that our time with the child is short and she can help by giving us a broader picture of his entire behavior. We treat the teacher with respect and try to show her that her views and observations of behavior are important to us. Our respect will get the teacher talking.

Along with the child's basic behavior we need information on his stuttering. Once again we begin with the general question letting her talk freely about the child's stuttering.

Of course, if we conduct the interview in this open-ended way the teacher will ask questions. One of the questions they usually ask concerns the cause of stuttering. "Did the parents do something to cause Johnny to stutter?" "Isn't stuttering a psychological or emotional problem?"

To these questions we might answer: "I'm not sure at this point what Johnny's home situation is like but it has been our experience that these stuttering children can come from almost any type of home environment. So we usually don't put all the blame on the parents. And we don't feel comfortable calling stuttering simply an emotional problem. Some children, it is true, seem to have a strong emotional base to their stuttering. The stuttering really is a way of showing us that they are not happy and that all is not well with their environment. However, many others seem to be quite well adjusted emotionally and the stuttering seems to be more of a developmental or learning problem. Some children have trouble with fine motor coordination and speech is a most difficult fine motor skill. These children develop problems speaking fluently. Usually they grow out of this disfluent period but some of them begin learning bad speech habits. They become worried or concerned about their stuttering or perhaps their parents have reacted negatively to their stuttering. Whatever the case the child begins trying too hard to speak fluently and as a result he starts having more trouble. That is one of the reasons for this meeting, we are trying to discover some of the causes of Johnny's stuttering."

This type of reply hopefully shows the teacher that her input is important. She is made to feel a part of the remediation process. As a result we should expect more cooperation from her in the future. She will be more willing to give up some of her break time to help us with our client.

Teachers will also want advice on how they should react to the child in the classroom. "Sometimes the other children laugh when Johnny stutters. I feel that I should do something but stuttering embarrasses me a little too."

To this we might answer: "And that's just the trouble with stuttering, you see. So many of us are ashamed and embarrassed by stuttering that little Johnny also begins to feel these negative emotions. What do you do when one of the children makes a mistake on a math problem and everyone laughs? You probably treat the situation quite casually and matter of factly so that the child won't feel as much pain and he will be willing to try again sometime. So to with stuttering. Treat the incident objectively. You might say something like this: 'Sometimes it's hard for Johnny to say some of his words but we will always listen to what he has to say'. Speaking directly and plainly will help not only Johnny but also the other children will feel less inclined to laugh next time. Now I know sometimes that's difficult and hard to do. Having a stutterer in your room is not the easiest experience but Johnny can really benefit by your understanding."

Or they may ask something like this: "Why is it that some days he's so fluent and then other days he can hardly talk?"

To this popular question our reply can include a suggestion for helping to manage the child's stuttering. "Stuttering does seem to be cyclical in nature. Perhaps this is no different than the rest of us when we talk about our good or bad days. We can do a lot to help Johnny if you can recognize these changes in his stuttering. On his fluent days you might encourage his class participation, calling on him more often than usual. One of the best ways of helping him talk more fluently is to give him good fluency experiences. So on good days give him many opportunities to speak so that he can feel the joy and satisfaction of talking fluently. Conversely on his bad days call on other children first. Of course, if his is the only hand up then sometimes you have no choice, but try to discourage his volunteering if possible. I'm sure your teaching experience will enable you to do this without his becoming suspicious."

As with parents we try to be careful about giving them a lot of don'ts but sometimes we need to change some of their behavior as this common question illustrates: "Well, you know, sometimes he gets stuttering so bad on a word that I say it for him. Is this all right? He doesn't seem to mind."

We must be careful in our reply not to condemn or criticize the teacher. "Sometimes you surely want to help Johnny, don't you? He's struggling so and the other children are getting nervous and you want to save him some embarrassment. But what we must consider is how will our reactions influence the child. If we do help him on a word, then perhaps he will begin to lose confidence in his ability to speak. How embarrassing to have someone help you with a word. Children can begin to lose their self respect and feel weakened by this. Or he might feel that his stuttering is bad since people cannot bear to let him finish. This only makes him try harder to speak perfectly and as a result, he stutters more. So even though our intentions were honorable and loving they may have had a negative effect on the child."

Teachers often ask us about how much verbal activity to demand from a stutterer. "Should I make him give his book report in front of the class like the others or can his be written and handed in? I hate to force him to talk if he is really embarrassed about it but yet what do I say to the other children?"

This is a difficult question and one with no clear cut solution. On the one hand forcing a stutterer to embarrass and humiliate himself seems wrong but at the same time if we grant him a special privilege then he will be ostracized by some of his peers and he may lose much in the way of confidence and self respect. We try to share this dilemma with the teacher. She should know how difficult this question is and hopefully help us make these everyday decisions. After discussing the pros and cons of the problem we might say:

"We usually recommend that the child be treated as normally as possible. After all school is meant to train children for adult life and Johnny will not be given special privileges as an adult. The world is often cruel and children need to deal with these realities. However, if you think that Johnny will fail miserably there is no sense in forcing him to give the report. Perhaps the best solution would be to ask him to stay a minute after school. You might say something like this: 'I wanted to talk with you about your oral book report. You have been having a lot of trouble talking and I wanted to know whether you were willing to give your report? It won't be easy and I wouldn't blame you for not wanting to give it. I won't penalize you for not giving the report but if you want to give it I would like you to. Why don't you tell me in the morning what you have decided. At that time you might tell me if you want to be the first one called on. Sometimes it helps to get it over with. Or perhaps you could raise your hand when you felt ready'. This little talk can really help you know and understand Johnny's feelings and he will feel like you genuinely care about him."

That would be one way to approach the problem of an oral report. Another way of dealing with this question is to call a meeting with both child and teacher. Each situation is so unique that if possible we should sit down with all the participants and work out an acceptable solution. We would also encourage the parents to attend. Everyone should not only be kept informed but should also feel that they are influencing the decisions. There are no simple answers to this problem of class participation so it is advisable to get as much input as possible in the decision making.

Other teachers have described a totally different problem. "I have been told that I should let Johnny talk as much as possible because we don't want him to feel that we are discriminating against him. But he has always got his hand up and when he starts talking you can't shut him up."

This is a common complaint with young stutterers in the early grades. We might say something like:

"That is a problem that other teachers have talked about. The child seems to be afraid that if he stops he might not be able to

start up again or he may have a need to talk in order to prove to himself that he's not afraid. Possibly he doesn't get enough chance at home so he makes up for it in school. Whatever the reason, once again we feel it is important to treat Johnny as normally as possible. If the other children don't get to talk that often then his output should be limited. Certainly you will probably want to bend the rules a little for Johnny but he shouldn't be allowed to dominate. After he has made a point and is beginning to go on to another you can stop him and restate his contribution in your own words. This shows him that you have gotten the message and felt it was important enough to repeat to the class. After repeating his contribution you might ask others to comment or add to what he said. In this way you have been able to stop him but yet he is left feeling that he has made an important contribution. But if he should attempt to continue then you can tell him that you have appreciated his comments but now someone else needs a turn."

In general we have found the best policy with teachers is to help them understand the problem of stuttering. This understanding often brings on the changes which will help our client. In addition to this information on stuttering we attempt to have them see their actions through the eyes of the stutterer. If they were in his shoes how would they feel? For some teachers this type of identification is valuable in their relations with the child. We attempt to show them how the stutterer feels when he is pitied or treated like a younger child. Or how difficult the classroom is for him when the teacher is very demanding and highly inflexible. We see through his eyes the falseness of a teacher who completely ignores his stuttering. He feels like an untouchable, that he is committing the great unmentionable. This creates a highly tense situation when the teacher ignores and refuses to face reality.

What the teacher needs to do is talk matter of factly with the child about his stuttering. She needs to let him know that she is aware of the stuttering and willing to help him make her classroom as pleasant as possible for him. Clinician, child and teacher will meet together and work as a team. This direct confrontation helps clear the air of misunderstood intentions. Understanding is the basis for our advice to teachers, parents and for that matter the entire therapy process for stutterers. We are convinced that like the iceberg the dangerous portion of the stuttering problem lies beneath the surface. The more we can expose to the light of reason and understanding the better the chance for the child to succeed This is the core of our belief and the reason for our success.

Concluding Remarks

The ideas described in this book have been the result of five years work with stutterers in the public schools. During that time we have seen over hundreds of young stutterers in our county-wide program. Although we haven't helped all of them to our satisfaction, we have never to our knowledge caused a stutterer to get worse.

Looking back over these five years we have learned much and gained valuable experience with stuttering children. Each year we learn more, and perhaps five years from now we will want to change or add to some of the material in this book. Our therapy changes as we learn more about the needs of our clients.

At the end of every year we have looked back to evaluate our program and have listed the major areas of emphasis that we felt were most important. At the top of the list each year is an admonition to get these stutterers into therapy at an earlier age. We are convinced that the younger we can identify the stutterer the better. If we can see these stutterers while they are still mild and relatively unscathed by their stuttering, then our involvement need not be a major one in terms of time and effort. And the prognosis for these young children is excellent. What a difference when compared to the long term therapy commitment of a severe, confirmed young stutterer who at best has a rather cloudy prognosis for future fluency. We are convinced that the vast majority of stutterers in grades 3 and above could have been worked with more successfully and with much less effort at an earlier age.

Most of us unfortunately have been taught to wait until stuttering has a firm foothold before we begin therapy. This seems so illogical. Other speech disorders are not treated this way nor for that matter are other physical or emotional problems in children. Certainly common sense tells us it is easier to tackle a problem at its onset.

But enough! We feel uncomfortable in the role of evangelist for our joy has come in the challenge and excitement of the therapy process. We have little interest in arguing the merits of certain methodologies for we are sure others have found success with stutterers using a variety of methods. Fine! Let's pool our information and see if we can't make some improvement in our treatment of the young stutterer.